Mediterranean Diet for Beginners 2024

The Upgrade Guide of Mediterranean Diet | Get Started on Your Wellness Journey with Easy, Quick, Healthy Recipes and Expert Nutrition Advice

Table Of Contents:

Introduction

Many people find it challenging to maintain a diet that is nutritious, healthy, and balanced. This difficulty often stems from poor food choices and unhealthy eating habits that are prevalent in our fast-paced modern lifestyle. Consuming highly processed foods, making poor diet decisions, and not being aware of healthy eating patterns can lead to an increased risk of chronic diseases such as type-2 diabetes, obesity, and heart disease.

The Mediterranean diet is a balanced approach to nutrition that emphasizes the consumption of whole, unprocessed foods and incorporates fundamental principles that promote optimal health. This diet primarily encourages the intake of foods like whole grains, fresh fruits, vegetables, seeds, nuts, and legumes, which are all rich in essential vitamins, minerals, fiber, and antioxidants. These nutrients are crucial for overall health and can help reduce the risk of chronic diseases. The diet plan is carefully designed to provide a balanced mix of essential nutrients, including proteins, fats, and carbohydrates, along with a variety of other necessary nutrients. A typical Mediterranean meal consists of a generous serving of vegetables, lean protein from fish, poultry, legumes, or eggs, whole grains, and healthy fats from seeds, nuts, and olive oil.

If you're ready to leave behind your unhealthy lifestyle and embrace a healthier one, our Mediterranean Diet Cookbook is your ultimate guide. This cookbook will help you understand the principles, scientific basis, and nutritional value of the Mediterranean diet. Learn how this time-tested dietary pattern can help improve your overall health, prevent chronic diseases, and enhance your well-being.

Our cookbook contains a wide range of delicious Mediterranean recipes, from breakfasts, appetizers, and snacks to vibrant salads, main dishes, side dishes, and desserts. These recipes are designed to satisfy your taste buds while providing plenty of essential nutrients. The cookbook also includes easy-to-follow meal plans to help you transition to the Mediterranean diet. Say goodbye to confusion and hello to nourishing meals that will energize and satisfy you.

The Mediterranean diet stands out from other diet plans because it's a sustainable approach to weight management that focuses on consuming wholesome, nutrient-dense foods. Our Mediterranean cookbook gives you the tools and knowledge you need to achieve and maintain a healthy weight without sacrificing taste. Adopting the Mediterranean diet can provide long-term health benefits. After switching to a Mediterranean-style eating pattern, you can expect increased energy levels, improved heart health, better digestion, enhanced brain function, and a greater sense of well-being. The diet has shown promising results in preventing and managing type 2 diabetes by focusing on low-glycemic foods like vegetables, whole grains, and legumes that help regulate blood sugar levels and improve insulin sensitivity. The diet also includes healthy fats and moderate alcohol consumption, which may contribute to better glycemic control.

The Mediterranean diet is one of the most researched, with numerous studies supporting its many health benefits. Here are a few examples of scientific studies that highlight the positive outcomes associated with the Mediterranean diet:

- The PREDIMED Study: This trial involved over 7,000 participants in Spain and examined the effects of adding extra-virgin olive oil or nuts to the Mediterranean diet. The study found that those who followed the Mediterranean diet had a lower risk of cardiovascular diseases compared to those on a low-fat diet.

- The PREDIMED-Plus Study: This clinical research project built upon the original PREDIMED trial's findings to investigate the effects of the Mediterranean diet on cardiovascular health in individuals at high risk due to obesity. The study found that participants who followed the Mediterranean diet, along with calorie restrictions and physical activity, improved their overall body weight, lipid profile, and blood pressure compared to the control group.

- The MIND Diet Study: Researchers at Rush University Medical Center conducted this study to investigate the effects of the MIND diet on cognitive decline and the risk of Alzheimer's disease. The study involved over 900 participants and found that the MIND diet helps reduce the risk of developing diseases like Alzheimer's.

- The Lyon Diet Heart Study: This study was conducted in France to examine the effects of a Mediterranean diet on cardiovascular disease. More than 600 people who had previously experienced heart attacks participated in the study. The study found that those who followed the Mediterranean diet had lower rates of recurrent heart attacks and a reduced overall mortality rate compared to those who did not.

These studies, along with many others, provide scientific evidence supporting the health benefits of the Mediterranean diet. Remember, the sooner you start this journey, the sooner you'll reap the amazing benefits of the Mediterranean diet. Don't let regret and missed opportunities hold you back. If you're ready to explore the world of the Mediterranean diet and unlock its life-changing secrets, don't wait another second. Dive into our Mediterranean Diet Cookbook and let the magic begin. Keep reading to discover the health secrets that await you. Your transformative adventure is about to start!

Chapter 1: Mediterranean Diet

What is the Mediterranean Diet?

The Mediterranean diet is a highly nutritious eating pattern based on traditional food preparation methods used by people living in countries along the Mediterranean Sea, including France, Italy, Greece, Spain, Turkey, Egypt, and Lebanon. This diet offers a broad range of balanced foods and is one of the most affordable, emphasizing seasonal plant-based foods like fresh fruits, vegetables, nuts, beans, whole grains, fish, and olive oil. It also permits moderate protein consumption and low dairy intake.

The Mediterranean diet restricts highly processed foods, artificial sweeteners, and processed meats. These foods are rich in essential vitamins, fibers, minerals, nutrients, and have antioxidant properties. The diet limits red meat intake and encourages moderate fish consumption, preferably cooked in olive oil. Fish is preferred due to its omega-3 fatty acids, which are beneficial for heart health and can lower the risk of heart attacks, type-2 diabetes, and even some cancers. The focus on whole foods and healthy fats in the Mediterranean diet can also aid in weight loss.

Mediterranean diet history

The Mediterranean diet is one of the oldest eating patterns and comes from the dietary habits of people living around the Mediterranean Sea, situated between Asia, Africa, and Europe. Its roots can be traced back to ancient civilizations like the Romans, Greeks, Egyptians, and others. Ancient Roman and Greek philosophers' historical records highlight the importance of the Mediterranean diet, known for its rich variety of seasonal fresh foods and numerous health benefits. The Mediterranean region has also been influenced by Moorish and Arab cultures, introducing new ingredients like citrus fruits, rice, almonds, and spices such as saffron, cumin, and cinnamon.

The Mediterranean region is renowned for its perfect climate and soil conditions for olive cultivation. Almost 90 percent of the world's olives are produced in Mediterranean countries like Greece, Italy, Spain, Tunisia, and Turkey. Thanks to their mild climate, seasonal fruits and vegetables are available year-round. As these regions are located along the Mediterranean Sea, fish is a staple in the diet, and fishing is a common occupation.

The Mediterranean diet goes beyond just the food consumed. It emphasizes the importance of sharing meals with loved ones, fostering a sense of community. This social aspect enhances the overall enjoyment of the Mediterranean diet and promotes a positive relationship with food. The Mediterranean diet has received considerable attention and praise from medical professionals and researchers for its numerous health benefits.

Exploring the Science of the Mediterranean Diet

The Mediterranean diet, inspired by the traditional eating habits of countries surrounding the Mediterranean Sea, is one of the most extensively studied nutritional plans. Research has consistently shown that this diet offers significant cardiovascular benefits, reducing the risk of heart-related diseases, including strokes and heart attacks, in both men and women.

The Lyon Diet Heart Study, conducted in France, investigated the impact of the Mediterranean diet on cardiovascular disease. The study involved over 600 participants who had previously suffered heart attacks. They were randomly assigned to either a Mediterranean diet group or a control group. The results showed that those following the Mediterranean diet had fewer recurrent heart attacks and a lower overall mortality rate than the control group.

The Mediterranean diet supplies our bodies with essential nutrients derived from fresh fruits, vegetables, seeds, nuts, whole grains, and legumes. These foods are rich in vitamins, minerals, fiber, and antioxidants, improving bodily functions and reducing the risk of chronic diseases.

Olive oil, the primary fat source in the Mediterranean diet, is rich in monounsaturated fats. These fats decrease LDL cholesterol levels and increase HDL cholesterol (good cholesterol) levels. They also improve insulin sensitivity and blood sugar control, reducing the risk of diabetes. Additionally, scientific evidence suggests that following the Mediterranean diet may be associated with a lower risk of breast and stomach cancer in women.

Advantages of the Mediterranean Diet

The Mediterranean diet, deeply rooted in the culture of Mediterranean countries for centuries, is one of the world's oldest and most trusted healthy eating patterns. This diet, more than just a food plan, offers numerous health benefits, including:

- **Enhanced heart health:**

The Mediterranean diet, with olive oil as its primary fat source, is rich in heart-healthy monounsaturated fats. These fats increase HDL levels and decrease LDL levels, improving overall cholesterol levels and reducing heart disease risk. The diet also encourages the consumption of fatty fish like salmon, sardines, and mackerel, rich in omega fatty acids. These acids improve blood vessel functions, reduce triglyceride levels, and have anti-inflammatory properties, reducing oxidative stress and cardiovascular disease risk.

- **Lowered risk of chronic disease:**

The Mediterranean diet, focusing on whole grains, legumes, fresh fruits, vegetables, and healthy fats, can help regulate blood sugar levels, improve insulin sensitivity, and reduce diabetes risk. Combined with regular exercise, the diet supports weight management efforts, helping to maintain a healthy weight. The diet's high intake of whole grains, fresh fruits, vegetables, and olive oil has anti-inflammatory and antioxidant properties, reducing the risk of developing colorectal cancer and protecting against neurological disorders.

- **Longevity:**

People in Mediterranean regions tend to live longer due to their healthy eating habits, physical activity, clean environment, and access to fresh foods. These foods, rich in antioxidants, combat the aging process and reduce the risk of chronic diseases, contributing to a healthier, longer life.

- **Better vision:**

The Mediterranean diet, rich in fresh fruits, vegetables, and whole foods, provides a high intake of antioxidants like vitamins C and E, zeaxanthin, and lutein, protecting the eyes against oxidative damage and reducing the risk of eye diseases.

- **Improved brain health:**

The Mediterranean diet, emphasizing antioxidant-rich fruits, vegetables, whole grains, nuts, and healthy fats, protects against inflammation, oxidative stress, and brain cell damage. The diet is linked to better cognitive function, including attention, memory, and executive function. It also supports brain health by improving cardiovascular health, maintaining blood vessels, and ensuring proper blood flow and oxygen supply to the brain.

Tips for Starting the Mediterranean Diet

- Increase your intake of plant-based foods: Start incorporating a wider variety of plant-based foods into your daily diet. This includes fresh fruits, vegetables, whole grains, seeds, legumes, and nuts. Aim to fill half of your plate with these nutrient-rich foods.

- Opt for healthy fats: Choose healthier fat options such as olive oil, avocados, nuts, and seeds, instead of unhealthy saturated and trans fats. Use olive oil as your primary cooking oil and consider using extra virgin olive oil for drizzling over vegetables and as a salad dressing.

- Prioritize fresh and seasonal food: Seasonal foods offer superior taste and flavor. They are readily available and can be preserved for longer periods. Whenever possible, opt for fresh and locally sourced ingredients to ensure you're getting the most nutrient-dense and flavorful produce.

- Reduce meat, increase fish: Incorporate fish and seafood into your diet, aiming for at least two to three servings per week. Fatty fish like salmon, mackerel, and sardines are excellent sources of omega-3 fatty acids, which are beneficial for heart and brain health.

- Cut back on red meat: Red meat is high in unhealthy saturated fat, which can increase the risk of heart disease and other cardiovascular conditions. Limit your red meat consumption, consider replacing it with fish or poultry, or switch to plant-based protein sources such as tofu, beans, and lentils.

- Experiment with herbs and spices: Use herbs and spices to add flavor to your meals without resorting to excessive sodium. Some recommended spices include smoked Spanish paprika, cayenne pepper, chipotle, and chili flakes.

- Exercise regularly: The Mediterranean lifestyle promotes regular physical activity. Aim for at least 150 minutes of moderate-intensity exercise per week to burn extra calories and build lean muscle mass.

Key Mediterranean Ingredients and Pantry Staples

- Olive Oil: This is a major component of the Mediterranean diet, prized for its high content of monounsaturated fats and antioxidants. It's used extensively in cooking, dressings, and dips. Olive oil also aids in lowering bad cholesterol (LDL) and raising good cholesterol (HDL).

- Fresh Fruits: These are packed with essential vitamins, minerals, and fiber. Mediterranean cuisine often includes fruits like apples, berries, figs, dates, grapes, peaches, oranges, grapefruits, pears, and melons.

- Vegetables: These nutrient-dense foods provide vitamins, minerals, fibers, and antioxidants. Commonly used vegetables in the Mediterranean diet include spinach, Brussels sprouts, kale, tomatoes, summer squash, onions, cauliflower, peppers, cucumbers, turnips, potatoes, sweet potatoes, and parsnips.

- Whole Grains: These are loaded with essential nutrients and dietary fiber, offering numerous health benefits. Whole grains such as wheat, rice, quinoa, barley, oats, rye, and brown rice are more nutrient-dense than refined grains. They are used to prepare dishes like whole wheat pasta, whole grain bread, couscous, and bulgur pilaf.

- Legumes: These are a great source of plant-based protein in the Mediterranean diet. Legumes like chickpeas, kidney beans, peas, fava beans, black beans, pinto beans, and lentils are low in fat and free of cholesterol, making them a healthier alternative to animal-based proteins.

- Nuts and Seeds: These are essential to the diet, providing plant-based protein. Healthy options include flax seeds, pumpkin seeds, sunflower seeds, sesame seeds, almonds, pistachios, hazelnuts, cashews, and walnuts.

- Fish and Seafood: These are rich in lean protein and omega-3 fatty acids, as well as essential nutrients, vitamins B and D, and minerals such as iodine, zinc, and selenium. Healthy choices include salmon, trout, clams, mackerel, sardines, tuna, and shrimp.

- Herbs and Spices: These are used to enhance the flavor and aroma of dishes in Mediterranean cuisine. Popular choices include oregano, mint, thyme, cinnamon, garlic, basil, nutmeg, rosemary, and parsley.

- Yogurt and Cheese: Both are good sources of calcium and protein. Yogurt also contains probiotics, which promote immune function, digestion, and overall health. Greek yogurt, skim milk, and low-fat cheese are popular in the Mediterranean diet, but goat cheese, feta cheese, and other varieties can also be used in moderation.

Chapter 2: The Mediterranean Way of Life

The Mediterranean Sea is surrounded by a diverse array of countries including but not limited to Italy, Morocco, France, Syria, Spain, Greece, and Egypt. Given the vast number of countries in this region, it's challenging to define a single diet that encompasses all their cuisines. However, the Mediterranean diet incorporates common elements from these areas such as a high intake of fruits and vegetables, whole grains, lentils, beans, fish and shellfish as an alternative to meat, and a generous use of olive oil. These elements form the core of the Mediterranean dietary regime.

The Philosophy Behind the Mediterranean Diet

The Mediterranean diet is more than just a passing diet trend, it's a lifestyle that has been embraced by millions of people living along the Mediterranean Sea for centuries. This lifestyle includes a variety of healthy, flavorful ingredients and a different approach to life compared to what most Americans are used to. The Mediterranean diet and lifestyle extend beyond just food, it also involves making small lifestyle changes that enhance your overall health quality.

Stress Reduction

In general, people residing in Mediterranean countries tend to experience less daily stress compared to Americans. They dedicate more time to enjoying meals with their loved ones and often take a brief nap after lunch. A common practice is a 2-hour midday break for lunch and a nap. Researchers who studied this post-lunch rest practice found that it significantly benefits health. Recent studies revealed that a regular short nap in the middle of the day can reduce the risk of death from heart disease by 37 percent!

The Impact of Stress

Often, doctors overlook the need to discuss the effects of chronic stress on long-term health during routine check-ups. This lack of information is unfortunate as stress might be the most significant health risk factor many of us face. Stress is challenging to measure in the same way we measure blood pressure or heart rate, making it somewhat elusive and subjective. What causes stress for one person might not for another. For instance, some people thrive under deadline pressures and fast-paced work environments, but might find the stress of starting a family overwhelming. Conversely, some people handle the daily pressures of raising children effortlessly, but could be overwhelmed by a fast-paced work environment.

Regardless of its source, chronic stress leads to an increase in cortisol and adrenaline, the stress hormones, which in turn raise blood pressure and heart rate, and increase the risk of blood clot formation. Studies have shown that individuals under chronic stress are more likely to suffer heart attacks. Additionally, highly reactive and impatient individuals are more susceptible to cardiovascular issues.

Regular Physical Activity

In addition to lower stress levels, regular physical activity is a common aspect of the Mediterranean lifestyle. People frequently walk, which is unsurprising given the beautiful weather and breathtaking views around the Mediterranean Sea. Whether it's an early morning stroll, walking to the grocery store, gardening, or sweeping the yard, physical activity is a natural part of life.

Family Bonding

Family plays a significant role in Mediterranean culture. Family gatherings are not just limited to holidays or special occasions, they occur every few days or at least once a week, fostering a strong bond among family members.

Chapter 3: The Mediterranean Diet in a Nutshell

The Mediterranean diet, characterized by its emphasis on whole, unprocessed foods and a diverse range of health-enhancing vitamins and nutrients, is widely acknowledged by health and dietary professionals as an optimal dietary approach for maintaining heart health and controlling weight. Its benefits have been proven in numerous clinical trials.

For many residents of the Mediterranean region, their dietary habits are not a diet, but rather a lifestyle that has been ingrained for thousands of years. This lifestyle includes consuming fresh, plant-based ingredients and engaging in regular physical activity.

There is no need to subscribe to pre-packaged Mediterranean diet meals or follow a specific calorie meal plan. No food group is off-limits, and carbohydrates are not to be avoided. Instead, the focus is on being more aware and thoughtful about daily eating habits, mirroring the approach of millions of people living along the Mediterranean Sea.

How the Mediterranean Diet Became Popular

The Mediterranean diet was first highlighted by American scientist Dr. Ancel Keys in the late 1950s. His Seven Countries Study examined the diet and lifestyle habits of participants from seven different countries: the Netherlands, Finland, Japan, former Yugoslavia, Italy, and the United States.

Keys' research revealed that dietary habits, types of fat intake, and physical activity significantly reduced the risk of cardiovascular disease among the study participants. Furthermore, it underscored that those who had already adopted this diet and lifestyle were residents of the Mediterranean region. Since Keys' study, hundreds of additional studies have been conducted, all reinforcing the numerous benefits of the Mediterranean diet. Chapter 3, "Who Should Consider the Mediterranean Diet and Why?" will delve deeper into Keys' research and other related studies.

While not every country bordering the Mediterranean Sea shares identical eating habits, most incorporate many elements of the Mediterranean diet into their culture and lifestyle. The specific foods consumed vary based on the country, culture, agricultural practices, and even regions within each country. This section of the book will help you understand the fundamental aspects of this diet.

Here are the key components that make this diet and lifestyle effective:

- Consumption of fresh, seasonal fruits and vegetables

- Minimization of processed foods

- Incorporation of whole grains into everyday recipes

- Utilization of "good" or unsaturated fats, sourced from fish, extra virgin olive oil, nuts, and avocados

- Moderate intake of low-fat dairy products like Greek yogurt, which is rich in probiotics beneficial for the digestive system, and cheese

- Consumption of lean proteins from eggs, fish, poultry, and small amounts of red meat

- Inclusion of legumes, such as beans, seeds, and nuts in the diet

- Use of fresh and dried herbs and spices for enhanced flavor

- Moderate consumption of red wine (optional for non-drinkers)

- Regular physical activity

- Stress reduction

- Spending quality time with family

While these are general guidelines, the most crucial point is to adapt each element in a way that suits your lifestyle, making it more likely for you to continue following these tips.

Creating a Mediterranean Table

Transitioning to a Mediterranean diet can be a significant shift, especially if you're used to the typical American eating habits. The Mediterranean diet emphasizes smaller portions and reduced meat consumption. Unlike the traditional main course and side dishes, Mediterranean meals often consist of several equally important dishes. Here are some guidelines to help you integrate this diet into your daily life.

Rethinking Your Meal Structure

Normally, you might choose a protein as the central part of your meal, with a few vegetable or starch dishes on the side. Instead, consider starting with one or two vegetables and make the protein a co-star, not the star of the show. This doesn't mean you'll be preparing more food; it simply requires a different approach to meal composition.

Importance of Portion Control

No matter what foods you eat, it's crucial to keep an eye on portion sizes. The Mediterranean diet typically involves smaller portions, as reflected in the recipes in this book. For example, you might be used to serving four people with a pound of pasta, but in this diet, you should aim to serve at least six. Also, a serving of chicken or meat should be around five ounces. Unfortunately, you won't find a 10-ounce steak in this diet! A Mediterranean meal consists of several dishes, each contributing a reasonable portion size.

Prioritizing Fresh and Local Produce

A significant part of Mediterranean meal planning is increasing the intake of vegetables and fruits. This diet also encourages eating seasonal produce to ensure freshness. While canned and frozen vegetables like fava beans, corn, tomatoes, and artichoke hearts are available all year round, fresh and in-season produce is preferable.

The Mediterranean diet largely avoids processed foods, focusing instead on dishes rich in flavor and low in preservatives and sodium. Seasoning comes from herbs and spices rather than unhealthy ingredients. This ancient diet harks back to a time when people ate what was in season, which is beneficial as in-season produce is more nutrient-rich.

Purchasing local produce also guarantees the freshest ingredients. Fruits and vegetables lose nutrients over time, so buying locally ensures you're getting freshly harvested produce packed with nutrients. When fresh produce isn't available, Mediterranean cultures have learned to preserve food without excessive salt, sugar, or fat, through drying and pickling.

A key aspect of the Mediterranean diet is that while about 35% of your calories come from fat, it's primarily from healthy monounsaturated fats found in olive oil, nuts, avocados, and fish. Nuts are a significant part of the diet, contributing to your protein intake. Including a handful of nuts daily can increase your intake of protein, omega-3 fatty acids, healthy fats, vitamin E, and fiber, while reducing cholesterol.

Incorporating Whole Grains and Legumes into Daily Meals

People living in the Mediterranean region often consume less red meat and poultry, instead, they get their protein from beans, lentils, nuts, and whole grains. These ingredients can be used in a variety of dishes like soups, stews, and salads. They can also be paired with protein sources like fish to make a meal more satisfying. Additionally, these components can be used to enhance pasta or vegetable dishes. While whole grains are a good source of essential nutrients such as antioxidants, it's important to note that not all grains consumed in the Mediterranean diet are whole grains.

Opting for Seafood Over Red Meat

The Mediterranean diet emphasizes the consumption of fresh fish and shellfish, a tradition that has been followed by the people living along the Mediterranean Sea for centuries. Seafood is beneficial for its low-calorie content and high levels of heart-healthy polyunsaturated fats. Affordable options of fresh fish include sardines and mackerel. There are numerous healthy ways to prepare fish, such as pan-roasting, broiling, grilling, and baking.

Utilizing Meat as a Flavor Enhancer

In the Mediterranean region, red meat is often expensive, hence it's commonly used in combination with more affordable ingredients like beans or grains, reducing the overall meat consumption. People following this diet often prepare dishes that accentuate meat along with a primary vegetable or grain. They tend to use more flavorful cuts of meat, so even a small amount can greatly enhance the taste of the dish.

Choosing Fruit Over Sweets for Dessert

In the Mediterranean diet, fruits are usually served as dessert, while cakes and cookies are reserved for special occasions. To reduce saturated fat intake, consider substituting part or all of the butter in your desserts with olive oil. However, to maintain a satisfying taste, you might need to keep some butter in the recipe. This might require some experimentation as you transition to this healthier eating and living style.

Embracing Variety in Meals

Mediterranean meals are known for their diversity, so experiment with dishes that offer a range of temperatures and flavors. The practice of serving some foods cold can simplify meal planning as these dishes can be prepared in advance or served as leftovers. As you explore more dishes that align with this dietary plan, you'll find it easy to interchange recipes.

The Mediterranean Diet Pyramid

The Mediterranean Diet Pyramid was developed in the 1990s as a joint effort between the nonprofit health and cultural food organization known as 'Oldways' and the Harvard School of Medicine. This visual guide was created in 1993 to depict the Mediterranean diet, providing a useful reference for those interested in adopting this eating plan. The pyramid essentially encapsulates the findings of Ancel Keys' Seven Countries Study. One of his key discoveries was that the inhabitants of Crete had lower heart disease rates than other participants in the study, a fact he attributed to their diet rich in vegetables, grains, and legumes, and low in saturated fat. The Mediterranean Diet Pyramid played a significant role in popularizing this diet in the United States. In 2008, the pyramid underwent minor revisions to produce the version described here.

Similar to the USDA food pyramid from the 1990s, the Mediterranean Diet Pyramid uses varying sizes of sections to indicate the relative importance of different food types in the diet. The base of the pyramid, representing the most frequently consumed foods, includes herbs and spices, nuts, olive oil, fruits and vegetables, whole grains, legumes, and beans. It is advised that those following this diet should center their meals around these base foods.

The next level of the pyramid features seafood, with a recommendation to consume fish and shellfish at least twice a week. Moving up, you'll find poultry, eggs, and dairy products, which should be eaten in moderation, either daily or weekly. At the top of the pyramid are red meats and sweets, which should be consumed sparingly and infrequently.

Red wine is also included in the diet, typically depicted on the side of the pyramid or in a small section beneath meats and sweets. Moderate consumption is recommended, usually defined as one to two 5-ounce glasses per day.

The pyramid also highlights the importance of hydration, reminding us to drink plenty of water. While water is not usually featured in food pyramids, it is a crucial part of any diet and lifestyle. Drinking water is especially important during exercise, as it aids metabolism. It's recommended to drink plain water instead of sugary sodas or fruit drinks, which often contain high fructose corn syrup. If plain water isn't appealing, try adding fresh fruit or herbs for flavor.

Lastly, most versions of the pyramid include a base section dedicated to the key elements of the Mediterranean lifestyle: daily physical activity, shared meals, relaxation, and abstaining from smoking.

Recommended Servings and Serving Sizes

The Mediterranean diet pyramid doesn't provide specific information about the recommended servings and serving sizes for each food group. However, dietary experts have provided some guidance on this matter. Here's an overview of how much you should consume from each food group and what a serving size looks like:

- Whole Grains: Aim for four to six servings daily.

A serving is equivalent to ½ cup of cooked grains like oats, quinoa, or pasta, or 1 slice of bread.

- Vegetables: Four to eight servings are recommended daily.

A serving is 1 cup of raw or ½ cup of cooked vegetables.

- Fruits: Consume two to four servings daily.

A serving is ½ cup of fresh fruit, 1 average piece of fruit, or ¼ cup dried fruit.

- Beans and Legumes: One to three servings are suggested daily.

A serving is 1/3 cup dried or 1 cup cooked.

- Seafood: Have two to three servings weekly.

A serving is 4 to 6 ounces.

- Fats: Three to six servings are recommended daily.

A serving is 1 ounce of nuts or seeds (the number varies depending on the size) or 2 tablespoons of nut or seed butter. For oils, a serving is one tablespoon.

- Herbs/Spices/Condiments: Use herbs generously. For condiments, aim for one tablespoon per serving. Limit salt to 1 to 2 teaspoons daily.

- Poultry: One to three servings are suggested weekly.

A serving is 3 to 4 ounces (approximately the size of your palm).

- Red Meat: Limit consumption to three to four servings monthly.

A serving is 3 ounces.

- Eggs: Three to four servings are recommended weekly (but egg whites can be consumed daily).

A serving is 1 whole egg.

- Dairy: Have one to three servings daily.

A serving is 1 cup of yogurt or 1 ounce of cheese; opt for low-fat or nonfat versions.

- Alcohol: Limit to one to two drinks daily.

A serving is 4 ounces of wine or 12 ounces of beer.

- Sweets: Avoid these and choose a serving of fruit instead.

For food groups with a range of servings, consider your body size and activity level. If you're a tall, muscular individual who's physically active, you can aim for the upper limits of serving sizes. Conversely, if you're smaller, less active, or aiming to lose weight, try to consume the lower number of recommended servings. For more information about weight loss, refer to Chapter 5: "The Mediterranean Diet and Weight Loss."

Chapter 4: Who Should Consider the Mediterranean Diet and Why?

This section explores the numerous health advantages associated with the Mediterranean Diet. If you find these benefits appealing or think that this diet could help with a specific health issue you're dealing with, it would be a good idea to discuss this dietary approach with your doctor.

Let's begin by examining the key components of the Mediterranean Diet and their primary health benefits!

The Main Parts and Health Benefits of the Mediterranean Diet

Whole Grains

Whole grains play a crucial role in the Mediterranean diet. Studies have proven that their consumption can reduce the risk of life-threatening conditions like diabetes, cancer, and heart disease. A single whole grain kernel is made up of an outer layer (the bran, which is rich in fiber), a middle layer (packed with complex carbohydrates and protein), and an inner layer (filled with vitamins, minerals, and protein). The process of refining grains, which is common in the United States, leaves only the middle layer intact, thereby eliminating the most nutritious layers. This results in grains that lack the disease-fighting vitamins and fiber. Examples of whole grains that can be incorporated into this diet include kasha, barley, oatmeal, and farro.

Whole grains, rich in fiber, vitamins, minerals, and complex carbohydrates, offer numerous health benefits. They aid digestion, lower cholesterol levels, help with weight loss by keeping you satiated for longer, and help prevent deadly chronic diseases related to poor cardiovascular health and high blood sugar levels. Whole grains are particularly beneficial for diabetics as they help regulate blood insulin levels.

Fresh Fruits and Vegetables

Farmers' Markets in the Mediterranean region are usually brimming with fresh, seasonal, locally-grown fruits and vegetables. These natural foods are rich in vitamins, minerals, complex carbohydrates, and fiber, helping to reduce the risk of cancer and heart disease, among other health issues. Phytonutrients, found in high quantities in the skins of these plant products, are powerful compounds that help combat serious health problems.

Incorporating fruits into your daily diet is quite simple. You can opt for easily portable fruits like apples, bananas, peaches, or apricots. Dried fruits are another excellent choice. They are convenient to carry, have a long shelf life, offer a concentrated flavor, and retain most of their nutrients. Fruits can also be added to your meals. Consider adding dried fruits or pomegranate to salads, enhance the taste of chicken with figs or dates, or add fresh fruit to Greek yogurt for a protein-rich, nutrient-dense snack!

Fruits also contain natural sugars, which are easier for your body to digest and are more nutrient-rich than refined sugars. These natural sugars, often referred to as fructose, are essential for the body, despite the negative connotations often associated with the word "sugar".

Moving on to vegetables, these nutrient-dense foods form another fundamental part of the Mediterranean diet. Vegetables are packed with fiber, vitamins, minerals, chlorophyll, potassium, carotenoids, flavonoids, and antioxidants. They are also low in fat, sodium, and cholesterol. In the Mediterranean diet, vegetables should form the foundation of every meal and occupy half of your plate. They are very low in calories, making them a beneficial dietary choice – they'll satiate you with all the right nutrients, without any unnecessary extras!

Nuts

Nuts such as walnuts, pine nuts, and almonds are delicious and packed with monounsaturated fat, which is beneficial for heart health. They are a staple in the Mediterranean diet due to their high fiber and protein content, which can aid in weight loss by promoting a feeling of fullness. Nuts also provide essential vitamins and have been linked to lower risks of heart disease, heart attacks, and high cholesterol. Their fiber and antioxidant content also support digestive health and slow down cellular aging. However, because they are calorie-dense, it's important to consume them in moderation. Also, avoid adding salt, sugar, or chocolate to maintain their health benefits.

Beans (Legumes)

Beans are another key component of the Mediterranean diet. They are rich in fiber, which can help reduce cholesterol levels and increase feelings of fullness. Beans also provide a good source of protein and vitamins. Regular consumption of beans has been linked to a lower risk of serious health conditions like heart disease, cancer, and diabetes.

Fish

Oily fish, common in the Mediterranean diet, are excellent sources of protein and omega-3 fatty acids. The omega-3 fatty acids in fish can positively affect cholesterol and triglyceride levels, reduce inflammation, and lower the risk of heart attack and sudden death from cardiac arrhythmias.

The two types of omega-3 fatty acids found in fish are EPA and DHA. EPA helps prevent blood clotting and reduce pain and swelling, and it can help manage heart disease, Alzheimer's disease, personality disorders, depression, high blood pressure, and diabetes. DHA supports brain function, blood thinning, and lower triglyceride levels, and it can help reduce the risk of type 2 diabetes, heart disease, dementia, and ADHD.

However, certain fish species may contain high levels of mercury and other contaminants. Pregnant women and young children should be cautious, but for most adults, the benefits of fish consumption outweigh the risks. Choose fish with low mercury levels like salmon, albacore tuna, herring, sardines, shad, trout, flounder, and pollock, and avoid fish like swordfish, shark, king mackerel, and tilefish, which typically have high mercury content.

Olive Oil

Olive oil, extracted from crushed and pressed olives, is central to the Mediterranean diet. It contributes to the unique flavor of Mediterranean cuisine and offers numerous health benefits. Olive oil is a monounsaturated fat that promotes heart health and contains polyphenols, antioxidants, and omega-3 fatty acids. These nutrients can help lower cholesterol and reduce the risk of diseases like cancer, heart disease, arthritis, osteoporosis, and type-2 diabetes.

Replacing butter or margarine with olive oil can reduce your risk of heart disease, inflammatory disorders, cancer, and diabetes. It can also help lower bad (LDL) cholesterol levels while maintaining or improving good (HDL) cholesterol levels.

A study in Boston showed that a diet rich in nuts and olive oil led to sustained weight loss over a year and a half compared to a low-fat diet. People also adhered to this diet longer due to the satiety provided by these foods.

Red Wine

Moderate consumption of alcohol, particularly red wine, can reduce the risk of heart disease. Red wine contains polyphenols and resveratrol, both of which support heart health. Resveratrol is an antioxidant that helps maintain healthy cholesterol levels and aids in blood clotting. It is found in higher quantities in red wine than white.

However, it's important to consume alcohol in moderation. Daily wine consumption should not exceed one or two 5-ounce glasses. For those who prefer not to drink wine, purple grape juice is a great alternative as it also significantly reduces the risk of heart attack.

Target Health Conditions of this Diet

The Mediterranean diet can potentially benefit various health conditions, some of which may not have been mentioned earlier. Here are some diseases or health issues that could be mitigated or even prevented by adhering to a Mediterranean-style diet:

- Cancer
- Depression
- Dementia
- Diabetes
- High Blood Pressure/Stroke
- Heart Disease
- Metabolic Syndrome
- Obesity

A Closer Look at Heart Disease

Often, discussions about the Mediterranean diet revolve around its potential to prevent heart disease and enhance heart health. This is primarily because cardiovascular disease is the leading cause of death globally. Let's examine the eight most common causes of death in the U.S. in 2010:

Heart disease: 600,000 deaths

Cancer: 575,000 deaths

Chronic lower respiratory diseases: 140,000 deaths

Stroke: 130,000 deaths

Accidents: 120,000 deaths

Alzheimer's disease: 85,000 deaths

Diabetes: 70,000 deaths

Kidney disease: 50,000 deaths

At first glance, heart disease and cancer fatalities appear similar. However, when considering deaths from cardiovascular disease – which includes heart disease but also impacts the entire circulatory system – the number rises to over 800,000. This encompasses heart disease, stroke (90 percent of which are clot-related and connected to the same process causing heart attacks), and various other conditions related to blood vessels. Diseases like diabetes, Alzheimer's, and kidney disease are also believed to be connected to or exacerbated by cardiovascular disease. Cancer ranks second, with approximately 575,000 deaths. Of these, 160,000 are due to lung cancer, primarily caused by smoking. The next most common cancers are colorectal (50,000 deaths per year), breast (40,000), pancreatic (40,000), and prostate (30,000). Each of these cancers can be caused by a mix of factors – such as genetics, diet, environmental toxins, hormones, and various carcinogens. In contrast, cardiovascular disease has a more singular cause, making its prevention plan potentially beneficial for a wider population. Moreover, the dietary and lifestyle guidelines that can help prevent heart and cardiovascular disease can also generally help protect against cancer – and all other major chronic diseases.

A History of Research Behind the Mediterranean Diet

The search for the perfect diet intensified in the 1940s when heart attacks started to rise at a worrying pace. Heart disease was the most pressing health issue at the time, accounting for approximately 40% of all deaths in the United States. This figure rose to 50% when stroke, a related condition, was included. The overall mortality rate was also higher, with arterial diseases causing about half of all deaths. This led to a significant number of people, in the prime of their lives, succumbing to sudden cardiac death. The situation reached a critical point when President Dwight Eisenhower suffered a major heart attack at 65 while still in office, leaving the nation anxious and in search of solutions.

Research projects and clinical trials independently conducted and widely publicized eventually revealed that the Mediterranean diet could be beneficial for individuals with cardiovascular disease and other conditions. Let's examine some of these studies:

The Seven Countries Study

Referenced earlier in the Mediterranean Food Pyramid's description, this pivotal twenty-year study by Dr. Ancel Keys established a connection between a diet low in saturated animal fat and processed food and a reduced mortality rate from coronary heart disease and cancer. Although diet had been suspected as a potential cause of heart disease since the beginning of the century, the link was still unclear. Cholesterol was considered a likely factor as it was found in abundance in arterial clots. When several significant studies showed higher cholesterol levels in patients with heart disease, many believed they had identified the dietary offender. However, Keys' studies revealed that dietary cholesterol was not responsible for the cholesterol found in the blood that could cause arterial blockages.

Keys started to theorize about other potential dietary factors causing high cholesterol levels when an unusual case pointed him in a new direction. A sick farmer was referred to him by a Wisconsin medical school. After various treatments, Keys checked the farmer's blood cholesterol level, which was extremely high - 1,000 mg/dL, compared to the national average of 220 or 230. The farmer's brother, who accompanied him, also had a high reading of 600. The brothers were sent to Keys' Minnesota lab, where they were put on an almost fat-free diet for a week. Their cholesterol levels dropped by about 50% after a week. Keys then decided to reintroduce fat into their diet. When they consumed food with saturated fat, their cholesterol levels shot up, suggesting that fat was influencing their cholesterol levels. This study led Keys to further investigate the impact of various types of fats on health and disease.

Keys continued to conduct additional feeding studies, which confirmed his belief that dietary fat intake influenced blood cholesterol levels. Post-war statistics offered another interesting clue. Keys observed that some of the wealthiest and presumably well-fed individuals in America had significantly high rates of heart disease. However, in post-war Europe, where food supplies like meat and dairy were scarce, heart disease rates had decreased. He was also intrigued by the reportedly low rates of heart disease in the Mediterranean region. Eventually, he moved to Italy in 1952 at the invitation of an Italian colleague.

Keys' research in Italy marked the beginning of international health and nutrition data collection for comparative purposes. He quickly noticed that cholesterol levels in Naples were significantly lower than those in America and England. Additionally, he observed that heart disease was uncommon in Italy during his hospital visits. Keys expanded his research to include Madrid, Spain, and his findings inspired an international team to gather similar data in South Africa, Japan, and Finland.

The collected data suggested a correlation between dietary fats, blood cholesterol levels, and the prevalence of heart disease. For instance, in Japan, communities with low heart disease rates consumed a low-fat diet. In contrast, in Finland, despite appearing physically fit, many men who consumed a diet rich in butter and cheese suffered from heart disease.

While in Naples, Keys became fascinated with the local food and culture. He appreciated the residents' culinary preferences, their active lifestyles, and their habit of enjoying a glass or two of wine with dinner. He discovered that the local diet was rich in fruits, vegetables, and whole grains, with less emphasis on dairy, meat, and sweet desserts. These observations led to the development of the Seven Countries Study.

The study, conducted with the help of renowned cardiologist Paul Dudley White, was a thorough ten-year investigation into the epidemiology of coronary disease in sixteen populations across six Western countries and Japan. Approximately 13,000 men aged between forty and fifty-nine from Japan, Greece, the Netherlands, Finland, Yugoslavia, and Italy were studied. The project, which began in 1958 after years of planning and fundraising, was a landmark study as it was the first to compare diet-disease associations across different cultures and lifestyles. The goal was to measure regional differences in risk, health behavior, and biological factors to provide guidance on preventing or slowing down heart disease worldwide.

The initial results of the Seven Countries Study, published in 1970, confirmed Keys' hypothesis that a diet high in fat, particularly saturated fat, was linked to heart disease. The island of Crete in Greece and southern Italy stood out in the study, having the lowest rates of heart disease and the longest life expectancy. In contrast, Americans had a 72% higher risk of dying from heart disease than Italians. The study found a clear link between diet and health, but the specific foods in the diets were not published immediately as the analysis focused on macronutrient contents (proteins, carbohydrates, and fats).

The Seven Countries Study sparked interest in the dietary habits of the world's healthiest people. Subsequent research highlighted the benefits of other aspects of the Mediterranean diet beyond low saturated fat intake. It was found that the antioxidants, vitamins, minerals, fiber, healthy proteins, complex carbohydrates, and wine consumed by these populations also contributed to their health and longevity.

Throughout the 80s and 90s, numerous experts including doctors, scientists, and nutritionists endeavored to pinpoint the exact definition of the Mediterranean diet. This was a challenging task given the diverse cuisines of the over fifteen countries bordering the Mediterranean Sea. However, they continuously found themselves referring back to the 1960s rural diets of southern Italy and Crete.

In 1989, a director involved in the Seven Countries Study released a historical account of the diets of the subjects in all countries involved in the study. The dietary proportions of southern Italy and Crete during that period are now considered the ideal healthy Mediterranean diet due to the extremely low prevalence of diet-related conditions in these communities at that time (though their diets and disease rates have since evolved). Other studies corroborated these findings, forming the primary research basis for the food proportions in contemporary Mediterranean diet pyramids.

The Lyon Diet Heart Study was one of the first clinical trials that supported the therapeutic benefits of the Mediterranean diet. Conducted in 1994, this revolutionary study involved 600 French heart attack patients who were randomly assigned to either a Mediterranean-style diet or a control diet similar to the one recommended by the American Heart Association for heart disease risk reduction. Two years into the study, the results were striking: the Mediterranean diet group had a 73% lower risk of coronary events and a 70% lower overall mortality rate compared to the control diet group. The study, originally intended to last five years, was halted early due to the significant beneficial effects observed in the Mediterranean diet group. Interestingly, despite the strong correlation between adherence to the Mediterranean diet and longevity, no significant associations were observed for the individual components of the diet. This suggested that the overall diet, rather than its individual components, was key to health and disease prevention.

Subsequent research revealed that the Mediterranean diet was beneficial not just for heart health, but also for any condition related to arteries or veins. A series of studies also demonstrated that adherence to the Mediterranean diet could lower the risk of various cancers and degenerative brain diseases such as Parkinson's and Alzheimer's. Furthermore, the Mediterranean diet has been widely acknowledged to reduce overall mortality.

Below are summaries of several other scientific studies that have contributed to the evidence supporting the numerous health benefits of the Mediterranean diet:

The DART Study: This study involved over 2,000 men and investigated whether the polyunsaturated fat in seafood could protect against heart disease. The results indicated that consuming a moderate serving of oily fish twice a week could reduce the risk of death from heart disease by 32% and overall mortality by 29%.

The Alzheimer's Disease Study: Dr. Nikolaos Scarmeas from Columbia University Medical Center in New York demonstrated a 68% lower risk of developing Alzheimer's disease with adherence to a Mediterranean diet. He also led another study showing that a Mediterranean diet could help Alzheimer's patients live longer, healthier lives post-diagnosis.

The Singh Indo-Mediterranean Diet Study: This trial involved 499 heart disease risk patients who were put on a plant-based diet. The study found that this dietary change reduced heart attack incidences and sudden cardiac death. The subjects also experienced fewer cardiovascular events compared to those on a conventional diet.

The Metabolic Syndrome Study: Dr. Katherine Esposito and her Italian colleagues examined the effects of a Mediterranean diet on patients with metabolic syndrome (a condition characterized by obesity, high blood pressure, unhealthy cholesterol levels, and signs of vascular inflammation). The Mediterranean diet improved all symptoms of metabolic syndrome.

The Study in Spain

A study conducted in Spain compared the effects of a Mediterranean diet to a low-fat diet. Although the study was initially planned to run for a longer duration, it was abruptly halted after only 4.8 years due to the remarkable results it yielded. Those who adhered to the Mediterranean diet experienced a substantial 30 percent decrease in major cardiovascular events, such as heart attacks, strokes, and death. On March 2, 2013, the New York Times reported that medical experts had declared that a diet had been proven for the first time in history to be as effective as medication in preventing cardiovascular complications, including death.

Recent Perspectives on the Mediterranean Diet

Around the year 2000, the fat content in the Mediterranean diet was scrutinized, challenging the long-held belief that a low-fat diet was the healthiest option. It was recognized that even though a diet high in fat was linked to heart disease, the regions that the Mediterranean diet was modeled after actually consumed a high-fat diet, with about 40 percent of their daily calories coming from fat. However, the type of fat they consumed was not saturated fat, but olive oil. Olive oil, rich in monounsaturated fat and antioxidants that offer numerous health benefits, seemed to be a crucial health potion, helping to prevent various diseases.

In 2005, an interdisciplinary, multicultural conference was held in Rome to further refine and standardize the Mediterranean diet. The participants introduced the ancient Greek term, ataraxia, meaning "equilibrium," "lifestyle," and a state of profound tranquility surrounded by trustworthy and loving friends, to describe the Mediterranean diet. They emphasized that the Mediterranean diet is more than just about food; it also involves a lifestyle that significantly impacts health and well-being. Physical, social, and culinary activities also play a vital role.

Despite extensive research, scientists have yet to discover a one-size-fits-all solution for health, likely because our bodies are too complex for such a solution. However, we seem to have pinpointed the diet of the people who suffer the least from diseases and live the longest. Perhaps the magic lies in the fact that the Mediterranean diet enhances universal biological characteristics that promote health, such as reducing inflammation and excess body fat. Or maybe it's the warm social environment that the healthiest communities enjoy. Or perhaps it's the simplicity, variety, and deliciousness of a diet so fresh that makes it easy to adopt. Most likely, it's a combination of all these factors.

Who Should Consider Switching to the Mediterranean Diet?

The Mediterranean diet is recommended for anyone seeking optimal cardiovascular health and wanting to prevent diet or lifestyle-related health complications. In essence, health experts widely endorse this diet as beneficial for almost everyone.

Potential Socioeconomic Barriers

However, a 2017 study suggested that the benefits of the Mediterranean diet might be more pronounced among individuals of higher income or socioeconomic status, or those with higher education levels. The study found that the heart health benefits of this diet seemed to be more significant among these groups.

The reasons behind these findings could be varied. It could be that higher-quality food, more readily available to wealthier individuals, contributes to the diet's benefits. Also, a wider range of food choices might be accessible to those with higher incomes. Lastly, it's plausible that those with more education could adhere more strictly to the diet and report their adherence more accurately. However, due to various factors influencing how people report their dietary habits, the accuracy of this research may not be entirely reliable.

Does this mean that those with lower incomes or less education should abandon the idea of benefiting from the Mediterranean diet? Absolutely not! It merely suggests that commitment to the diet is crucial for everyone, regardless of income, background, or education level, to enjoy its benefits. The key is making consistent, small steps towards improvement.

Moreover, those with lower incomes might face greater challenges in sourcing high-quality ingredients. However, it's still feasible to follow the Mediterranean diet on a tight budget. Generally, whole, unprocessed foods are cheaper than processed ones. Fresh fruits and vegetables, especially local produce, are typically affordable. Canned light tuna in water is as beneficial as fresh salmon. There are also many cost-effective whole grains, and poultry is usually budget-friendly. Since the diet includes limited quantities of red meat and dairy, these items shouldn't strain your budget too much.

Regarding pricier items like olive oil, herbs, and spices, it's recommended to buy these in small quantities to prevent spoilage. The next chapter will introduce the most commonly used spices and herbs, giving you a starting point. It's also advised to start with only what you need for your initial recipes and gradually build your pantry from there. There's even a buying guide for olive oil!

People with Food Allergies and Intolerances

Yes, it's true that the Mediterranean diet has several elements that could potentially trigger allergic reactions in some individuals, such as certain nuts, shellfish, dairy, and gluten-containing products. However, even those with these allergies can adapt this diet to suit their needs!

If you're allergic to shellfish, dairy, or nuts, there are still numerous sources of protein and unsaturated fats in this diet. So, you can still adhere to it by making the appropriate replacements. If you're already used to making these dietary modifications, these adjustments shouldn't pose much of a challenge.

For those with gluten allergies or intolerances, the Mediterranean diet is still a viable option. A common misconception about the Mediterranean diet is that it heavily relies on bread and pasta. But as you've learned from this book, there are many other essential components of this diet that don't contain wheat or gluten at all. Furthermore, many whole grains are gluten-free, including amaranth, buckwheat, corn, millet, most whole oats, rice, sorghum, and wild rice.

Also, quinoa, while not technically a grain, can be eaten in a similar manner to grains and is gluten-free. If you've been diagnosed with a gluten intolerance, like Crohn's disease, or gluten sensitivity, you're probably already familiar with making gluten-free substitutions in your diet. So, don't worry, the Mediterranean diet is still accessible to you!

NOTE: Always Consult Your Doctor!

Regardless of your level of physical fitness, health issues, or food allergies, it's always highly recommended to seek advice from your healthcare provider before switching diets or starting a new workout routine. Your doctor can address any potential concerns that might require you to follow a specific version of the Mediterranean diet. They may also suggest that you undergo certain tests before making any dietary changes or after adhering to a new diet for a few months.

In the following chapter, we'll guide you on how to start incorporating the Mediterranean diet and mindset into your daily life.

Chapter 5: Getting Started

Adopting the Mediterranean diet can be a thrilling journey. The initial decision to enhance your diet and overall life quality is the first step towards this healthier lifestyle. It may seem daunting initially, but remember, you don't have to implement all changes at once. The more minor modifications you make, the more benefits you'll reap, motivating you to continue making positive changes. These benefits will yield significant long-term rewards for you and your family.

Keys to Embracing the Mediterranean Lifestyle

To successfully integrate this new dietary approach into your life, it's worth considering the adoption of other aspects of the Mediterranean lifestyle.

Manage Your Stress Levels

Recall the discussion on stress dangers in Chapter 1? One of the most crucial aspects of adjusting your lifestyle to align with your new dietary habits is stress management! This might be challenging since everyone experiences stress at different points in their lives. Moreover, some individuals seem to have more stressful lives than others. Regardless, managing stress should start by gaining a realistic understanding of what causes our stress, followed by efforts to change these factors. While you may not be able to adopt the Mediterranean habit of a 2-hour midday break, you can find ways to reduce your stress throughout the day.

Firstly, a regular exercise routine can significantly aid in stress reduction. Research has shown that active individuals handle stress better. This is because regular aerobic exercise lowers adrenaline levels, which rise less dramatically during stressful situations.

Aim to engage in some physical activity every day. This can be as simple as walking your kids to the park or taking a 20-minute stroll with your dog while appreciating nature, instead of being glued to your phone. If physical activity isn't feasible, try making a cup of coffee or tea, disconnecting from technology, and spending 20 minutes relaxing on your porch. It's these small moments that allow your body and mind to rest.

Alongside regular exercise, relaxation techniques such as meditation, yoga, or self-hypnosis can also help lower your overall stress levels. If these lifestyle changes don't significantly reduce your stress, consider seeking professional help from a psychologist or psychiatrist.

Here are ten practices to try for stress reduction:

- Regular exercise
- Meditation
- Prayer
- Maintaining close relationships with friends and family
- Setting realistic life goals
- Living within your financial means
- Yoga
- Pursuing interests and hobbies outside of work
- Maintaining a positive outlook on life and keeping your sense of humor
- Laughing, smiling, and enjoying your life!

Engage in Regular Exercise

While we've previously discussed the importance of exercise for stress reduction, it's worth delving deeper into this topic. Regular physical activity is a key aspect of the Mediterranean lifestyle, and it offers benefits beyond stress management. Common forms of exercise in the Mediterranean region, such as walking to the market or gardening, are integral to maintaining good health. Regular exercise boosts good cholesterol (HDL), reduces blood pressure, and enhances bone health, thereby lowering the risk of osteoporosis. It also fosters a sense of well-being, which explains the abundance of healthy, happy seniors in the Mediterranean region.

The recent surge in obesity in America can be attributed to a lack of exercise and poor dietary choices. Numerous studies have indicated that physical unfitness can be more harmful to our health than simply being overweight. Unfortunately, we've become a nation of "couch potatoes," and encouraging people to adopt a regular exercise routine can be challenging. We prefer taking the elevator over the stairs, parking as close as possible to stores, and using carts instead of walking during a golf game.

The solution lies in integrating exercise into your daily routine. You don't need to start with strenuous activities like jogging 5 miles or cycling for an hour each day. A simple 30-minute walk daily can significantly reduce the risk of heart attacks and other cardiovascular issues. Moreover, a regular exercise regimen can decrease fatigue and enhance lung function. Incorporating light weight resistance training can further improve bone health and help maintain muscle tone.

It's your responsibility to identify a physical activity you enjoy, figure out how to incorporate it into your lifestyle, and stick with it until it becomes a habit. There are numerous ways to include exercise in your daily routine, such as walking during your lunch break, walking your kids to the park instead of driving, cycling on Saturday mornings instead of watching TV, walking between stores while shopping, or engaging in a sport that the whole family can enjoy. If you have kids, you can set a good example by showing them that physical activity is a crucial part of life.

Here are some additional simple tips to incorporate exercise into your daily routine:

- Walk in place for 30 minutes while watching TV.
- Park further away from your office or grocery store and take a short walk through the parking lot.
- Spend the first part of your lunch break walking before eating.
- Use a pedometer and aim for 10,000 steps daily.
- Opt for the stairs occasionally.

Physical activity is a crucial component of the Mediterranean diet. To successfully adopt this diet, you must incorporate exercise into your lifestyle along with making healthy food choices.

Spending Quality Time with Family

In this technologically advanced and fast-paced world, finding time for family can be challenging. However, it's crucial to prioritize family time. One way to do this is by scheduling shared meal times. This not only strengthens bonds but also fosters a sense of belonging. Studies have shown that strong family interactions can help reduce the risk of depression.

If you're not living close to your family, you can replicate this atmosphere with friends. Consider organizing weekly or bi-weekly gatherings, with a different friend hosting each time. Turning these gatherings into potluck meals can alleviate the pressure of meal preparation from one person. When you attend, bring along a recipe from the Mediterranean diet to share!

Additional Tips for Embracing the Mediterranean Lifestyle

Apart from reducing stress, increasing physical activity, and enhancing family time, here are some other guidelines to consider as you adopt the Mediterranean lifestyle. Remember, you don't have to make drastic changes all at once. You can start small and gradually incorporate these guidelines:

- Include a variety of fresh, whole foods in your diet.

- Minimize fat intake, except for healthy unsaturated fats.

- Avoid refined sugar.

- Reduce salt intake.

- Control portion sizes.

- Drink alcohol moderately, preferably red wine.

- Stay hydrated by drinking plenty of water.

- Maintain a positive attitude, laugh, smile, and enjoy life. Don't lose your sense of humor.

- Quit smoking. If you're a smoker, start taking steps to quit today.

- Take time to relax every day, especially after meals if possible.

A Fresh Look at Your Kitchen

It's crucial to keep your kitchen well-stocked when you're embracing a new diet. You don't want to find yourself with an empty pantry, with only unhealthy snacks like chips or pre-packaged cake mix to eat. Having a variety of healthy foods on hand will give you numerous options for meals. Don't forget to experiment with various herbs, spices, and flavors, as they can add a lot of taste to your dishes without adding calories or fat.

While the Mediterranean diet includes familiar foods like chicken, salmon, quinoa, and chickpeas, it's worth exploring less common ingredients and looking up recipes that use grains like barley, beans such as chickpeas, meats like oxtails, and unique seafood like monkfish. If you're really committed to this diet, you might want to learn how to use tricky ingredients like grape leaves and phyllo dough, and flavor enhancers like sumac, preserved lemons, and pomegranate molasses.

This book contains only 20 recipes, which is just the beginning of countless other healthy dishes that you can discover through research. Here's some information about essential kitchen ingredients you might want to start stocking up on. It's not advised to buy all the spices, herbs, condiments, and other long-lasting ingredients at once as it can be quite expensive! Instead, choose the recipes you want to try first and start your shopping list with the ingredients needed for those dishes. Over time, you'll find that your pantry and fridge are well-stocked with ingredients from each of the following categories:

Fresh Fruits and Vegetables

Fruits and vegetables make up a significant part of the Mediterranean diet food pyramid. It's best to buy these foods when they're in season for the best flavor. Buying produce in season, and as close to the time it was harvested, ensures you get fruits or vegetables with the most nutrients. One way to ensure you're getting fresh produce is to buy from local farms and farmers' markets. It's also a good idea to smell produce before you buy it. If it smells good, it's likely to taste good, too.

Key fruits in the Mediterranean diet include: Apples, apricots, avocados, bananas, berries, dates, figs, grapes, melons, olives, peaches, pomegranate, and strawberries.

Popular vegetables in this diet include: Artichokes, beets, bell peppers, carrots, cauliflower, dandelion greens, eggplants, garlic, leafy greens, onions, potatoes, romaine lettuce, tomatoes, and zucchini.

You might have noticed that tomatoes are listed as a vegetable. While technically a fruit, tomatoes are generally treated as a vegetable in cooking, hence their inclusion in the vegetable list. Tomatoes and tomato products play a significant role in the Mediterranean diet, from fresh tomatoes to tomato sauce, tomato paste, and more.

Many recipes in this book, and from the Mediterranean region, include garlic and onions. These two ingredients can add a lot of flavor to any dish. They're versatile and can be cooked in different ways to change their flavors and intensity. For instance, slow-sautéed onions have a sweet taste, and garlic toasted in olive oil has a nutty flavor. Both can also be used raw in salads or dressings.

The recipes also demonstrate how vegetables can be easily incorporated into dishes in a variety of ways. However, remember that vegetables are healthiest on their own, so avoid adding heavy creams or sauces that can increase the calorie and fat content. The more vegetables you consume, the more benefits your body reaps, so try to include them in your meals as much as possible.

Beans: Dried and Canned

In the Mediterranean diet, legumes are a staple source of protein, along with fruits, vegetables, and whole grains. Legumes, which include chickpeas, fava beans, lentils, peas, and white beans, can be consumed fresh or dried. They can be eaten on their own or incorporated into various recipes, such as whole-wheat spaghetti with lentils or shrimp with white beans.

Canned beans are ideal for salads, stir-fries, and soups, while dried beans are best for slow-cooked dishes like stews, where their flavor can fully develop. Some people prefer to brine dried beans to maintain their shape during cooking. Fava beans are unique in that they are often used fresh rather than dried or canned, although this requires more effort.

Legumes are cost-effective and have a long shelf life when dried, making them a common ingredient in Mediterranean countries, especially during winter when meat and vegetables are scarce. To rehydrate them, simply soak in water and cook as needed. They can also be cooked, frozen, and quickly defrosted for convenience, offering a healthier alternative to canned goods that may contain preservatives.

Grains

Grains, including rice, are a key component of many Mediterranean dishes. Each type of grain requires a different cooking method. For instance, farro needs to be boiled in plenty of water, while rice requires just enough water to be fully absorbed. Aim for at least half of your grain intake to be whole grains, as refined grains are less nutritious and can increase the risk of diseases like diabetes.

Whole grains, such as bulgar, corn, oats, barley, brown rice, buckwheat, farro, freekeh, spelt, wheat berries, whole rye, whole-wheat flour, and wheatberries, are incredibly versatile. Quinoa, a nutty-flavored seed, is also considered a whole grain due to its similar preparation and consumption methods. Whole grains can be used in soups, pilafs, baked goods, or as stuffing. For a healthier option, replace all-purpose flour with whole-wheat flour, long-grain rice with brown rice, and regular pasta with whole-wheat pasta.

Pasta and Couscous

Pasta is a fundamental ingredient in many Mediterranean dishes, often prepared in ways unfamiliar to most American home cooks. For example, some pasta dishes are flavored with potent spices like cinnamon or cloves. Whole-wheat pasta provides a hearty alternative to the typical pasta Americans are used to. Couscous, a staple in North Africa, is used in a variety of dishes or served on its own. In the eastern part of the region, pearl couscous, which has larger grains and is toasted rather than dried, is commonly used.

The Olive and Its Oil

Olives are a staple in Mediterranean cuisine. Various types are used to produce olive oil, while some are specifically cultivated for direct consumption. It is advisable to opt for olives found in the refrigerated section of your grocery store, as they are often superior in quality to those preserved in cans or jars, which can be excessively salty due to preservatives. If you have the time, it is recommended by culinary experts to buy olives with pits and remove them yourself.

More information about olive oil will be provided in a separate section of this chapter.

The Use of Fresh and Dried Herbs

Herbs and spices became an integral part of the Mediterranean diet pyramid in 2008 due to their importance in this diet. They enhance the taste of food without adding extra calories or fat, and also contribute vitamins and minerals to your meals. Moreover, they have a long shelf life; dried herbs and spices can retain their quality for a year or more if stored in airtight containers.

Recipes may call for either fresh or dried herbs, depending on the desired flavor. Fresh herbs tend to have a robust, earthy taste, while dried herbs have a more subdued, nutty flavor. Fresh herbs can be added directly to dishes, while dried herbs often need to be cooked to release their flavors.

Mediterranean dishes are often seasoned with a variety of fresh herbs like basil and mint. Many enthusiasts of this diet grow their own herbs, while others buy them from grocery stores or farmers' markets. In the recipes provided in this book, fresh herbs are used both as garnishes and as key flavor contributors. Fresh herbs have a limited shelf life, but with careful handling, they can be stored for about a week. After rinsing and drying them carefully, wrap them loosely in paper towels, then place them in a ziplock bag and store in the refrigerator.

It is also beneficial to have a variety of dried herbs on hand, as they are frequently used in Mediterranean recipes. Blends of different herbs can add a rich, complex flavor to dishes. Dried herbs tend to lose their flavor within a year of opening the container. To check for freshness, rub a small amount between your fingers and sniff for the herb's distinctive aroma. If the aroma is absent, discard the herb and replenish your stock. Some fresh herbs, such as rosemary and thyme, can be dried in a microwave.

Common herbs used in the Mediterranean diet include basil, bay leaf, cilantro, marjoram, mint, oregano, parsley, rosemary, sage, and thyme.

Mediterranean Cuisine and its Spices

Mediterranean cuisine is diverse and can be differentiated by the unique spices used in each region's recipes. Common spices like cinnamon and paprika might already be in your pantry, while others such as sumac and Aleppo pepper might be new to you. Mediterranean cooking also utilizes spice pastes and dry blends to infuse dishes with unique flavors. Some examples are za'atar, a popular blend from the eastern Mediterranean; ras el hanout from North Africa; and harissa, a North African chili paste. You can buy these blends from certain supermarkets or grocery stores. If they're not available, you can learn to make them yourself with some research and practice.

To prolong the shelf life of your spices, store them away from heat and light. Pay attention to their smell and appearance; if either changes, it's likely time to discard them. When purchasing spices, you might notice that higher-quality brands tend to be more expensive. However, the enhanced flavor they bring to your dishes often justifies the additional cost. Moreover, a small amount of spice can flavor many meals, making the cost per meal relatively low.

Common spices used in Mediterranean cooking include allspice, black pepper, cayenne, cinnamon, cloves, coriander, cumin, dried ginger, paprika, sumac, and zaatar.

Salt

Salt is a key ingredient in maximizing the flavor of a dish, which is why almost every recipe in this book calls for it. You can use common table salt or opt for sea salt, which contains more minerals and is less processed. Don't be concerned about the sodium content in these recipes. The small amounts of salt used only minimally increase sodium levels. The high sodium levels harmful to cardiovascular health are typically found in processed foods, which contain large amounts of salt-based preservatives to extend their shelf life.

Cheeses, Cured Meats, and Nuts

Small amounts of cheese (like feta), cured meats (like pancetta), or nuts can significantly enhance the flavor of Mediterranean dishes. For instance, a little salami or prosciutto can add a lot of flavor to some dishes, while a sprinkle of Parmesan cheese can complete the taste of many pasta and salad dishes.

Nuts are a staple in the Mediterranean diet. They're delicious on their own or as part of sweet or savory dishes. Whether they're roasted, toasted, or raw, nuts like walnuts, pine nuts, almonds, pistachios, sesame seeds, peanuts, and cashews are packed with flavor. They're often added to salads and side dishes. Some spice blends also include nuts as a key ingredient. Some recipes in this book will show you how to easily incorporate nuts into your diet.

Despite the recommended dairy intake being only two servings per day, it's best to choose low-fat options as dairy products are high in saturated fat. Avoid processed cheeses and opt for fresh cheese made from sheep's or goat's milk. These are usually more flavorful, and a small amount can go a long way.

When storing cheese in the refrigerator for more than a few days, wrap it in parchment paper first to allow it to breathe, then in aluminum foil to prevent it from drying out and absorbing other flavors from the fridge. For long-term storage of nuts, keep them in the freezer to prevent them from becoming rancid. To enhance the flavor of nuts in recipes, try toasting them in the microwave or on the stovetop before adding them to dishes.

Fresh Meats, Poultry, Eggs, and Seafood

The Mediterranean diet is rich in a variety of meats like beef, lamb, poultry, eggs, and seafood, which offer essential proteins in moderate portions.

Traditional Mediterranean cuisine often includes beef, lamb, and goat, but these are consumed in moderation. When buying red meats, it's best to choose lean cuts. For example, fillet, though pricey, is an excellent choice due to its tenderness and low fat content. It can be grilled without adding extra fat and seasoned with fresh or dried herbs and spices for added flavor. For minced meat, whether beef or lamb, aim for a ratio of 95% lean meat to 5% fat. This small fat content helps retain moisture and flavor in the meat. Spices can further enhance the taste.

Poultry and eggs are also excellent protein sources. Chicken, duck, turkey, and other fowls are usually quite budget-friendly and can be cooked in various ways. To reduce saturated fat, remove the skin before cooking. For a leaner option, use the breast meat. It's recommended to have a 6- to 8-ounce serving of poultry every two days.

Eggs, despite their reputation for being high in fat and cholesterol, are actually recommended in the Mediterranean diet. You're encouraged to consume up to 7 eggs per week as they are a top source of high-quality protein and are relatively low in calories.

Seafood is a great alternative for those who aren't fans of poultry or red meat. It's high in protein, low in fat and calories, and packed with various vitamins and minerals. When buying seafood, it's best to choose fresh fish from a reputable source. Ideally, the seller should have a high turnover rate to ensure the fish hasn't been sitting in the display case for more than two days. If the fish has a foul odor, it's best to avoid it. Also, steer clear of cooked fish displayed next to raw ones to prevent cross-contamination. If fresh fish isn't available, frozen fish is a good alternative. However, make sure to cook it immediately after thawing.

Sauces and Spreads

Yogurt: You might find it surprising that yogurt is often used as a sauce or spread in the Mediterranean diet. It can be used as a topping or mixed into sauces and poured over various dishes. Some Mediterranean recipes call for the richer taste of full-fat yogurt, but low-fat or nonfat yogurt can be used in certain dishes. Greek yogurt, which is thicker and creamier than regular yogurt, is common in Mediterranean countries and worldwide. It contains live and active bacteria beneficial for your digestive and immune systems. Greek yogurt can be used as an ingredient or a side dish in many recipes for breakfast, lunch, or dinner. It's especially great for making the thick and creamy Tzatziki sauce, which can be used as a dip or sauce for dishes like kebabs, gyros, and falafel.

Tahini: This spread is made from ground sesame seeds and can be used as a topping on its own or mixed into sauces and dips, such as hummus and baba ghanoush.

Pomegranate Molasses: This thick, syrupy sauce, made by reducing pomegranate juice, is used to add a tangy flavor to many dishes. If you can't find it in stores, you can easily make it at home.

Preserved Lemons: This unique ingredient originates from North Africa. Preserved lemons are simple to make but take several weeks to cure. Once cured, they can be stored in the refrigerator for up to six months without spoiling. If necessary, you can make a quick substitute using lemon zest, lemon juice, water, sugar, and salt.

Dukkah: This Egyptian condiment is a mix of spices, seeds, and nuts used to add a unique flavor to various dishes. It can also be mixed with olive oil and used as a bread dip. As you become more familiar with Mediterranean cooking, you might prefer to make your own dukkah.

Honey: Honey is a natural sweetener excellent for use in baked goods, desserts, breakfast dishes, teas, and coffee. It contains 70 to 80 percent monosaccharides, fructose, and glucose, which give it its sweet taste. Research has shown that honey's antiseptic and antibacterial properties can help with colds or wound healing.

Flavored Waters: Have you ever tried orange blossom water or rose water? While they don't have significant nutritional value, they both have strong flavors and add an exotic taste to any dessert or drink. You can find them at specialty food stores at a reasonable price.

Syrups: Syrups in Mediterranean cooking are most commonly used as a dessert topping. Simple syrup, for example, is made by simmering sugar, water, a bit of lemon juice, and a flavoring such as orange blossom water or rose water. It can then be drizzled over phyllo pastries, fruit, or yogurt for added sweetness.

All About Olive Oil

Olive oil is a crucial element of Mediterranean cuisine. It's uniquely derived from the pressing and crushing of olives, making it a distinctive feature of this diet. The quality of olive oil is categorized into various grades, with "extra-virgin" being the highest. This grade is recommended for both cooking and raw uses in this diet plan. The flavor profile of olive oil can significantly vary based on the type of olives used and their ripeness at the time of harvest. While the Mediterranean region is renowned for its olive oil production, California also stands as a leading producer in North America.

Olive oil is known for its health benefits, particularly in promoting the intake of beneficial unsaturated fats. Substituting butter or margarine with olive oil can significantly improve heart health. As a plant-based food, it's packed with antioxidants and vital nutrients that aid in combating diseases such as cancer and diabetes.

Extra-virgin olive oil is a popular choice for dressings and as a delicious bread dip. Besides these common uses, it's also frequently used to enhance the flavor of vegetables and pasta, incorporated into meat and fish sauces, and used in the preparation of soups and stews. For a healthier dessert option, consider substituting butter with olive oil in pastries. For instance, an olive oil-based pie or tart crust can offer a delightful savory taste and delicate texture.

Choosing and Preserving Olive Oil

Selecting the right extra-virgin olive oil for your culinary needs can be a daunting task. Regrettably, the guidelines for olive oil quality are often optional and seldom implemented, meaning that bottles marked as "extra virgin" may actually contain a company's inferior olive oil, sold at an unjustifiably high price.

Extra virgin olive oils vary greatly in terms of price, color, and quality, making it challenging to decide which one to purchase. Several factors influence the style and taste of olive oil, the main ones being the type of olive used and the harvest time (with earlier harvests resulting in greener, more bitter, and stronger oils). Weather conditions and processing methods also play a role. The highest quality olive oil is derived from olives that are pressed as soon as possible without the use of heat. Although heating the olives during pressing extracts more oil, it compromises the exquisite flavor of the end product.

Given the wide array of extra virgin olive oils available in grocery stores, experts from America's Test Kitchen decided to simplify the selection process for consumers. They set out to identify the best "everyday" extra virgin olive oil and the best "luxury" product, with the aim of providing reliable product recommendations.

In their quest to find the best "everyday" olive oil, the testers sampled 10 budget-friendly olive oils in various dishes. They also sent each oil to a laboratory for quality and grading assessment. Additionally, they sought the opinions of 10 professional olive oil tasters on each variant.

In the end, one oil stood out among the rest: the California Olive Ranch Everyday Extra Virgin Olive Oil. The superior quality of this product was attributed to the company's meticulous control over every stage of production, from harvesting to bottling. Given that olives quickly lose their flavor after being picked, speed is crucial in the process of transforming them into oil and bottling it before it oxidizes and spoils. Priced at $9.99 for a 500 mL bottle, it is costlier than some subpar oils in the supermarket, but it is significantly more affordable than luxury oils.

Interestingly, the most expensive luxury oils are not necessarily the best. The luxury oil that received the highest rating from America's Test Kitchen is Gaea Fresh, a product from Greece. Priced at $18.99 for a 500 mL bottle, it is relatively affordable compared to other luxury olive oils. The tasters were particularly impressed by its robust yet well-rounded flavor. It is advised to use this luxury oil only in raw dishes, where the strong flavor is appreciated.

Of course, there are numerous other opinions on the best olive oil for your culinary needs. As you gain more experience with using and tasting olive oil, you might even discover your preferred brand of extra virgin olive oil. Don't hesitate to experiment and conduct your own research!

Maintaining the Freshness of Your Olive Oil

Three key factors can guide you in assessing the quality of extra-virgin olive oil before you buy it and in preserving its freshness.

Source of the Oil: Bottlers often indicate the origin of their oil on the label. Opt for oil that comes from a single country.

Harvest Date: Although some oils may have a "best before" date, the harvest date is a more reliable indicator of freshness. Generally, olive oil begins to deteriorate around 18 months after the olives are harvested. Aim to buy a bottle with the most recent date, ideally within the past year. If the harvest date is not provided, it might be best to avoid that bottle. Since olives are harvested in the fall and winter in the Northern Hemisphere, the bottles available might only list the previous year.

Packaging: Only dark glass effectively protects the oil from damage caused by light and air. Clear glass and plastic containers are not adequate for preserving the freshness and quality of your olive oil.

To Store

It's crucial not to leave your olive oil in a place where it's exposed to light. This is because olive oil, being derived from plants, contains chlorophyll which oxidizes when exposed to sunlight. Also, avoid storing your olive oil in places prone to high heat, like a cabinet next to the oven. The ideal storage place is a cool, dark cabinet. However, it should not be stored in the refrigerator as this will cause it to become thick and cloudy. Once a bottle of olive oil is opened, it should be used within three months. An unopened bottle, on the other hand, can be stored for up to a year.

To determine the freshness of your olive oil, all you need is your sense of smell. Pour a small amount and take a whiff. If it smells like stale walnuts or crayons, it's a sign that the oil has gone rancid and it's time to discard the bottle.

Now that you're equipped with this knowledge, you can start making necessary adjustments in your life. Specifically, if you're aiming to lose weight, it's time to explore how the Mediterranean diet can assist you in achieving your weight loss goals.

Chapter 6: The Mediterranean Diet and Weight Loss

The Mediterranean diet, which includes a balance of healthy fats and complex carbohydrates, is a superior option to trendy diets for those wanting to lose weight without compromising their health. Coupling this diet with less stress and more physical activity can result in more than just weight loss. It can also lower your blood pressure, cholesterol, and blood sugar levels. As discussed in previous chapters of this book, these are just the beginning of its benefits.

One of the primary ways diet impacts health is through weight management. Being overweight can harm every system in your body and puts you at risk for many severe and debilitating diseases. The Mediterranean diet aids in maintaining a healthy weight by offering complex carbohydrates, fiber, and protein, which help you feel full and slow down digestion, keeping you satisfied for longer.

The people residing in the Mediterranean region, who adhere to the Mediterranean diet and lifestyle, are generally slimmer than their American counterparts for several reasons:

• Physical activity is a regular part of their daily routine.

• Their diet includes high-fiber foods such as fruits, vegetables, beans, nuts, and whole grains, which contribute to a feeling of fullness.

• They steer clear of trans fats, which are linked to weight gain and obesity, opting instead for healthy fats like monounsaturated fat and omega-3 fat. These fats, found in olive oil, nuts, and fish, also help create a sense of fullness.

• They favor complex carbohydrates over simple ones and avoid refined sugars, which are associated with obesity. Complex carbohydrates also contribute to prolonged feelings of fullness.

• Unlike in America, food in Mediterranean countries is not typically served in large portions. It's the quality, not the quantity, of food that defines a good meal!

Calories and Weight Loss

The key to losing weight is straightforward: burn more calories than what you ingest. In essence, Americans are taking in too many calories! We have large meals and then snack while watching TV in the evening. This high calorie consumption, coupled with our inactive lifestyle, is why obesity is a major public health concern. While the Mediterranean diet isn't focused on rigorous calorie-counting, there are several strategies you can adopt to help you decrease your overall calorie intake, without needing to keep track of every calorie you consume.

Portion Control

We need to eat wisely. First off, we need to control the portions of food we consume. Over time, the size of restaurant meals and pre-packaged food portions have steadily increased. The average bagel now weighs four to five ounces (equivalent to four or five slices of bread), cookies are as big as saucers, and a restaurant pasta serving could once feed a family of four. To determine what a "normal" serving of pre-packaged food should be, check the nutrition label. You might be surprised to find out that the "single" pre-packaged food portion you thought was for one is actually meant for two – or more. You don't need to weigh or measure foods, just use common sense and learn to estimate correct portions. For example, a medium orange is about the size of a tennis ball, and a three-ounce piece of meat is about the size of your palm.

You learned about the recommended serving sizes and number of servings for each food group in the Mediterranean diet. As suggested in that chapter, you can use your body size, activity level, and weight loss objectives to determine the number of servings you should have within these guidelines. If you adhere to these recommendations, you might be able to lose weight without counting any calories. However, if you find it difficult to lose weight just by controlling portions and number of servings, you can learn more about counting calories later in this chapter.

Increased Physical Activity

In addition to controlling our portions, we also need to begin exercising. In chapter 4, you read several tips on gradually incorporating more physical activity into your life. If you lack motivation, remind yourself that you're doing this for more than just your waistline – regular exercise is crucial for a long and healthy life. By establishing and maintaining a daily exercise routine, you're ensuring that you'll be able to enjoy life with your loved ones for as long as possible.

Another tip to boost your exercise motivation is to find a partner who can help you stay accountable. Having a workout buddy not only assists you when you find it hard to get up and get moving, but it also adds elements of fun and social interaction to your exercise routine.

More Whole Foods, Fewer Processed Foods

Lastly, we also need to substitute processed foods, refined sugars, trans fats, and saturated fats with healthier, lower-calorie whole foods – as suggested in the Mediterranean diet. Also, because the focus is on fresh food, you're not consuming commercially-produced products that are higher in calories and designed to make you overeat and develop irresistible cravings. It's also easy to follow because it doesn't require a drastic diet overhaul, and – as you'll discover when you start trying recipes – it's delicious!

Counting Calories

The Mediterranean diet doesn't encourage strict calorie counting. Instead, it promotes the consumption of fresh, whole foods, controlled portion sizes, and avoidance of processed foods. Coupled with increased physical activity, this approach should naturally lead to weight loss. However, if you're stuck at a certain weight or hit a weight loss plateau, you might need to start counting calories until you can gauge your body's nutritional requirements.

Understanding Your Metabolic Needs

The first step in determining the number of calories you need to consume to lose weight is to calculate your basal metabolic rate (BMR). This is the amount of energy (in calories) your body would burn if you were to sleep all day. Here's how to calculate it:

1. Convert your height to centimeters. You can either measure it directly in centimeters or convert your height in inches by multiplying it by 2.54. For instance, if you're 63 inches tall, multiply that by 2.54 to get approximately 160 cm.

2. Convert your weight to kilograms. Take your weight in pounds and divide it by 2.2. For example, if you weigh 135 pounds, divide 135 by 2.2 to get about 61.4 kg.

3. If you're a man, calculate your BMR in calories per day using this formula:

BMR = (height in cm x 6.25) + (weight in kg x 9.99) - (age x 4.92) + 5.

4. If you're a woman, use this formula:

BMR = (height in cm x 6.25) + (weight in kg x 9.99) - (age x 4.92) - 161.

Next, calculate your total energy expenditure (TEE) per day, which is the amount of energy (in calories) your body burns each day based on your current activity level. Multiply your BMR by a factor that corresponds to your physical activity level (PAL) to get your TEE. Here's how:

• If you lead a sedentary lifestyle or engage in very light activity, like working in an office, multiply your BMR by 1.53.

• If you're active or moderately active, like doing house chores or getting a moderate amount of daily exercise, multiply your BMR by 1.76.

• If you're very active, with heavy physical labor or intense daily exercise, multiply your BMR by 2.25.

For instance, if a woman has a BMR of 1275.27 calories per day and leads a moderately active lifestyle, she would multiply 1275.27 by 1.76 to get approximately 2,244 calories. This is roughly the number of calories she needs to consume daily to maintain her current weight of 135 pounds.

Understanding Your Weight Loss Requirements

When aiming to shed pounds, the primary method is to consume fewer calories than you burn. This can be achieved in two ways - either by increasing your physical activity while maintaining your current caloric intake, or by reducing the number of calories you consume daily. You can also opt for a combination of both, but it's crucial to avoid making too many drastic changes. If you consume significantly fewer calories than your body requires, you could face serious health issues. In the worst-case scenario, your body could enter a "starvation mode," conserving every bit of energy to survive. In such a situation, you might not lose as much weight as you initially intended. The goal is to find a balance where you have a sufficient calorie deficit to lose weight while still providing your body with enough energy.

The safest way to figure out the number of calories to cut is by using simple mathematics. A sensible and safe weight loss strategy is to aim for a loss of 1 to 2 pounds per week. To lose one pound, you need a deficit of 3,500 calories. Spread over a week, this equates to a daily deficit of 500 calories. You can achieve this by either burning an additional 500 calories through exercise, consuming 500 fewer calories, or a combination of consuming 250 fewer calories and burning an additional 250 calories.

For instance, let's consider a woman who weighs 135 pounds and needs to consume 2,244 calories daily to maintain her weight. Suppose she wants to lose one pound per week until she reaches her target weight of 120 pounds. She has three options:

1. She can maintain her current activity level and consume 1,744 calories daily, creating a daily calorie deficit of 500.

2. She can engage in daily activities that burn an additional 500 calories while still consuming 2,244 calories daily.

3. She can consume 1,996 calories daily and engage in activities that burn an extra 250 calories daily.

With any of these three options, the woman will achieve a weekly calorie deficit of 3,500 calories, which should result in a weight loss of approximately one pound per week.

Assistance with Calorie Counting

Every recipe in this book provides an accurate calorie count per serving, along with protein, carbohydrates, and fat content. While this book only contains 20 recipes to get you started, you can find countless Mediterranean diet recipes online and in other books when you're ready to try more dishes. Many of these recipes will also include calorie counts.

If you want to try a recipe that doesn't provide calorie information, use your judgment and compare it to similar recipes. Alternatively, you can calculate the total calories of the entire recipe by adding up all the ingredients and dividing the total by the number of servings.

There are numerous mobile and tablet apps that can help you track your calorie intake and provide motivation when you achieve your daily goals. You can also search the internet for calorie counts of different foods and meals, often yielding surprisingly accurate results.

If You're Still Not Losing Weight - Problem Solving

Sometimes you might feel like you're doing everything correctly, but the weight just won't come off. Or maybe you initially lost weight quickly, but now you've hit the infamous plateau. If you find yourself in this situation, here are some strategies you could try:

- Seek medical advice. Your doctor might want to conduct blood tests to rule out any hidden metabolic issues.

- Alter your workout routine. Your body becomes more efficient at performing familiar exercises over time, meaning it burns fewer calories. By changing your workout, you "trick" your muscles into working harder and burning more energy.

- Increase your water intake. Your body metabolizes energy more effectively when it's properly hydrated. So, here's another reason to drink more water!

- Reduce your food intake slightly. Try eliminating one snack, one dessert, or half a side dish per day to see if a slightly larger deficit helps. Remember, don't take your calorie deficit to extremes!

- Eat a bit more. Your body might be too deprived and entering the so-called "starvation mode." Many people have found that by consuming an extra 200 healthy calories (lean protein, vegetables, fruit, or whole grains) each day, they were able to achieve their weight loss goals.

- Focus on enjoying your life, maintaining a healthy diet, and spending time with loved ones. Many people have found that when they concentrate on the positive aspects of life and stop obsessively counting calories, they gradually lose weight without much effort.

If you're still struggling with weight loss and nothing seems to work, it might be time to revisit your doctor or consult a registered dietitian (RD). These professionals can provide expert advice to help you fine-tune your diet and set you on the right path.

Eating Out on This Diet

Eating out can often pose challenges, regardless of the dietary regime or lifestyle you're adhering to. Many restaurant dishes are laden with salt, fat, and preservatives, making them unsuitable for consumption.

Nevertheless, it's still possible to enjoy a meal out while following the Mediterranean diet. Seek out eateries that cater to your health-conscious preferences, such as those offering fresh fruits and vegetables instead of deep-fried or sauce-heavy sides. Opt for dishes that aren't prepared using butter or rich sauces, and request for sauces or dressings to be served separately so you can regulate your intake.

These days, many restaurants provide calorie information for their dishes on the menu, aiding us in making healthier choices. If such information isn't provided on the menu, most chain restaurants make it available on their websites. Having this information beforehand can assist you in making an informed decision before you even reach the restaurant. This way, you're less likely to succumb to tempting offers or promotional specials upon your arrival at the restaurant.

Don't hesitate to ask your server for suggestions, or if they could inquire with the chef about making modifications for you. You could ask for a lighter dressing or request a dish to be grilled instead of fried. Remember, you're the customer, so don't shy away from politely requesting what you want.

Chapter 7: Recipes

Breakfast Recipes

Breakfast holds a significant place in the Mediterranean diet because it supplies the energy your body needs to carry out daily tasks and is regarded as a crucial meal. Although breakfast customs vary across the various regions and countries bordering the Mediterranean Sea, they generally reflect the dietary habits of this area. A Mediterranean breakfast is packed with fresh, whole foods, offering an ideal mix of nutrients.

Breakfast is the first meal you have after a long night of fasting. It's often recommended to have a nutritious breakfast as it supplies your body with the energy and nutrients it needs to jumpstart your metabolism, aiding both physical and mental activities. Breakfast provides vital nutrients such as vitamins, carbohydrates, proteins, and healthy fats. It sets the stage for the day by supplying the necessary fuel for physical and mental activities. A Mediterranean-style breakfast is a great source of complex carbohydrates from whole-grain foods, ensuring a steady energy release throughout the morning to prevent mid-morning energy dips.

The Mediterranean diet primarily encourages the consumption of healthy, nutrient-rich foods like whole grains, fresh fruits, vegetables, and healthy fats. Incorporating these nutrient-rich foods in your breakfast guarantees an early intake of essential vitamins, antioxidants, fiber, and minerals, enhancing your overall health. This diet offers a balanced approach to nutrition. Enjoy a balanced breakfast with a mix of nutrients like proteins, carbohydrates, and fats to keep your cravings in check and help maintain your blood sugar level. Mediterranean cultures strongly advocate the use of fresh, seasonal, and locally sourced healthy ingredients. Fresh fruits, vegetables, and other products are available for breakfast. It's often seen as a time for family or community gatherings, where people come together to share a meal. A nutritious breakfast can help manage your hunger and prevent overeating later in the day.

1- Greek Yogurt with Berries and Honey

This healthy dish takes 10 minutes to prepare and 5 minutes to cook, and it serves one person.

Ingredients:

- ¾ cup of Greek yogurt

- 1 tablespoon of honey

- 1 cup of fresh strawberries, chopped

- ½ cup of fresh blueberries

Instructions:

- Put Greek yogurt in a serving bowl.

- Place blueberries and chopped strawberries on top of the yogurt.

- Drizzle honey over the top and serve.

Nutritional Information (Per Serving):

- Calories: 151

- Fat: 0.7g

- Carbohydrates: 38.9g

- Sugar: 31.5g

- Protein: 1.6g

- Cholesterol: 0mg

2- Healthy Shakshuka

This nutritious dish takes 10 minutes to prepare and 25 minutes to cook, and it serves four people.

Ingredients:

- 4 eggs

- ½ teaspoon of smoked paprika

- 1 teaspoon of cumin

- 15 oz can of chopped tomatoes

- 1 tablespoon of harissa

- 1 marinated roasted red pepper

- 2 garlic cloves

- 1 tablespoon of olive oil

- Salt

Instructions:

- Heat oil in a pan over medium heat.

- Add garlic, harissa paste, cumin, tomatoes, roasted red peppers, paprika, and a pinch of salt, and cook for 5 minutes.

- Create four wells in the mixture and break eggs into them. Turn heat to low and simmer for 15-20 minutes or until egg whites are set, and egg yolk is runny.

- Garnish with freshly chopped parsley and serve.

Nutritional Information (Per Serving):

- Calories: 133

- Fat: 8.7g

- Carbohydrates: 8.1g

- Sugar: 5g

- Protein: 7g

- Cholesterol: 165mg

3- Avocado Toast

This dish takes 10 minutes to prepare and 5 minutes to cook, and it serves two people.

Ingredients:

- 2 slices of bread

- 2 tablespoons of crumbled feta cheese

- 2 tablespoons of fresh dill, chopped

- 2 tablespoons of pitted olives

- 1 ½ avocados, scoop out the flesh

- Pepper

- Salt

Instructions:

- Heat a pan over high heat.

- Add bread slices to the pan and cook for 1-2 minutes on each side. Remove bread slices from the pan and set aside.

- In a bowl, add avocado flesh and mash using a fork. Add cheese, dill, olives, pepper, and salt and mix until well combined.

- Spread avocado mixture onto bread slices and serve.

Nutritional Information (Per Serving):

- Calories: 374

- Fat: 32.7g

- Carbohydrates: 20.2g

- Sugar: 1.5g

- Protein: 5.6g

- Cholesterol: 8mg

4- Mediterranean Omelet

This dish takes 10 minutes to prepare and 10 minutes to cook, and it serves two people.

Ingredients:

- 5 eggs

- 2 teaspoons of avocado oil

- ¼ cup of sliced black olives

- ¼ cup of diced tomato

- 2 cups of chopped baby spinach

- ¼ cup of diced red bell pepper

- 2 teaspoons of olive oil

- Pepper

- Salt

Instructions:

- In a bowl, whisk eggs with pepper and salt. Set aside.

- Heat olive oil in a pan over medium-high heat.

- Add bell pepper and sauté for 2-3 minutes.

- Add olives, tomatoes, and spinach, and cook until spinach is wilted. Remove the pan from heat and set aside.

- Heat 1 teaspoon of avocado oil in a separate pan.

- Once the oil is hot, add half of the egg mixture to the pan and cook until the egg is completely set.

- Add half of the vegetable mixture to half of the omelet, then fold the omelet in half and slide it out of the pan.

- Repeat the same with the remaining egg and veggie mixture.

- Serve and enjoy.

Nutritional Information (Per Serving):

- Calories: 239

- Fat: 18.2g

- Carbohydrates: 5.3g

- Sugar: 2.3g

- Protein: 15.3g

- Cholesterol: 409mg

5-Overnight Oats Recipe

Prep Time: 5 minutes

Cook Time: 5 minutes

Serves: 1

Ingredients:

- Half a cup of oats

- 1 teaspoon of date molasses

- 1 teaspoon of tahini paste

- 2 tablespoons of chopped walnuts

- 4 tablespoons of yogurt

- 2 chopped dried figs

- 1 teaspoon of chia seeds

- A quarter teaspoon of ground cinnamon

- An eighth of a teaspoon of ground nutmeg

- Half a cup of almond milk

Instructions:

- Combine oats, figs, yogurt, almond milk, chia seeds, cinnamon, and nutmeg in a glass jar and mix thoroughly.

- Cover the jar and refrigerate it overnight.

- Before serving, top with walnuts and drizzle with date molasses and tahini paste.

- Enjoy your meal.

Nutrition Facts (Per Serving):

- Calories: 442

- Fat: 17.5 g

- Carbs: 60.5 g

- Sugar: 23.2 g

- Protein: 15.3 g

- Cholesterol: 4 mg

6-Fresh Fruit Salad Recipe

Prep Time: 10 minutes

Cook Time: 10 minutes

Serves: 6

Ingredients:

Dressing:

- 4 tablespoons of fresh orange juice
- Juice of 2 limes
- 2 tablespoons of honey

Salad:

- 1 cup of pomegranate arils
- 3 peeled and sliced kiwis
- 3 peeled and segmented oranges
- 2 cored and sliced pears
- 2 cored and sliced apples
- 8 chopped fresh mint leaves
- Half a cup of chopped walnuts

Instructions:

- Whisk together all the dressing ingredients in a small bowl and set it aside.
- In a large bowl, combine pomegranate arils, kiwis, oranges, pears, apples, and walnuts.
- Drizzle the salad with the dressing and toss to mix.
- Garnish with chopped mint and serve.

Nutrition Facts (Per Serving):

- Calories: 236
- Fat: 6.7 g
- Carbs: 45.1 g
- Sugar: 33.3 g

- Protein: 4.3 g

- Cholesterol: 0 mg

7-Smoked Salmon and Cream Cheese Bagel Recipe

Prep Time: 10 minutes

Cook Time: 10 minutes

Serves: 2

Ingredients:

- 2 halved and toasted bagels

- 1 cucumber, peeled into ribbons

- 1 tablespoon of chopped fresh dill

- 2 tablespoons of fresh lemon juice

- 4 ounces of cream cheese

- 4 ounces of sliced smoked salmon

- Pepper

- Salt

Instructions:

- In a small bowl, combine cream cheese, dill, lemon juice, pepper, and salt.

- Spread the cream cheese mixture on both halves of each toasted bagel.

- Layer cucumbers, salmon, onions, and capers on the bottom half of the bagels, then place the top half of the bagels on.

- Serve and enjoy.

Nutrition Facts (Per Serving):

- Calories: 564

- Fat: 24.3 g

- Carbs: 61.2 g

- Sugar: 8.2 g

- Protein: 26.6 g

- Cholesterol: 75 mg

8- Vegetable Frittata

Time to Prepare: 10 minutes

Time to Cook: 14 minutes

Serves: 6

Ingredients:

- 10 eggs

- ½ cup of crumbled feta cheese

- ¼ cup of diced green onions

- ½ cup of julienned sun-dried tomatoes

- ¼ cup of almond milk

- 3 cups of chopped kale

- ½ cup of sliced onion

- 1 tsp of olive oil

- 1 sliced fennel bulb

- Pepper

- Salt

Instructions:

- Set the oven to preheat at 400 0F.

- Heat oil in an oven-safe pan on medium-high heat.

- Add onion, fennel, and kale, then sauté for 5-7 minutes.

- In a bowl, whisk together eggs, almond milk, pepper, and salt. Mix in green onions and sun-dried tomatoes.

- Reduce the stove heat to medium, then pour the egg mixture into the pan. Press down the veggie mixture with a spatula.

- Sprinkle crumbled feta cheese on top and cook for an additional 5 minutes.

- Transfer the pan to the preheated oven and cook for 15 minutes.

- Cut into slices and serve.

Nutritional Information (Per Serving):

- Calories 204

- Fat 13.2 g

- Carbohydrates 9.8 g

- Sugar 2.3 g

- Protein 13 g

- Cholesterol 284 mg

9- Banana Pancakes

Time to Prepare: 10 minutes

Time to Cook: 10 minutes

Serves: 2

Ingredients:

- 3 eggs

- 2 ripe bananas

- ½ tsp of vanilla extract

- ¾ cup of rolled oats

Instructions:

- Combine eggs, bananas, vanilla, and oats in a blender and blend until the mixture is smooth.

- Spray a pan with cooking spray and heat it over medium heat for 30 seconds.

- Pour a spoonful of the batter onto the hot pan and cook until it's lightly golden brown on both sides.

- Serve and enjoy.

Nutritional Information (Per Serving):

- Calories 319

- Fat 9 g

- Carbohydrates 48.4 g

- Sugar 15.4 g

- Protein 13.6 g

- Cholesterol 246 mg

10- Green Smoothie Bowl

Time to Prepare: 10 minutes

Time to Cook: 5 minutes

Serves: 2

Ingredients:

- ½ of a ripe mango, peeled and chopped

- 1 cup of peeled and chopped pineapple

- 1 ripe banana, peeled and sliced

- 1 tsp of lime zest

- 1 tsp of fresh lime juice

- ½ tsp of vanilla

- 2 tbsp of honey

- ½ of an avocado, scoop out the flesh

- 2 cups of chopped fresh spinach

- 1 cup of almond milk

- For the topping:

- 4 sliced fresh strawberries

- ¼ cup of blueberries

- 1 tbsp of coconut flakes

Instructions:

- Add all the smoothie ingredients into the blender and blend until smooth.

- Pour the blended smoothie into two serving bowls and garnish with the toppings.

- Serve immediately and enjoy.

Nutritional Information (Per Serving):

- Calories 624

- Fat 40.1 g

- Carbohydrates 71.4 g

- Sugar 51.8 g

- Protein 6.8 g

- Cholesterol 0 mg

Appetizer and Snack Recipes

Mediterranean diet heavily relies on appetizers and snacks, which are integral to its overall eating pattern. These small servings allow for a diverse range of tastes, textures, and nutrients to be consumed throughout the day, encouraging mindful eating. The smaller portions also help in managing portion sizes, thus preventing overeating. This approach aids in maintaining a healthy body weight and avoiding excessive calorie intake by letting you savor different tastes without having to eat large amounts of food.

The Mediterranean diet's appetizers and snacks are a tasty and fulfilling way to incorporate plant-based ingredients into your diet. These wholesome ingredients are packed with essential vitamins, minerals, antioxidants, and fiber, which contribute to overall health improvement. Many of these appetizers and snacks feature antioxidant-rich ingredients like olives, artichokes, tomatoes, and herbs such as basil and oregano. These antioxidant-rich foods enhance your overall wellbeing and help ward off various diseases.

The Mediterranean diet's appetizers and snacks also foster mindful eating habits. Savoring a few almonds, a serving of fresh vegetables with dip, or a small dish of olives cultivates an awareness of tastes, textures, and hunger signals.

In terms of social and cultural aspects, meals are typically enjoyed leisurely, with appetizers often served before the main course. This practice encourages conversation, social interaction, and a relaxed approach to consuming healthy food. Many Mediterranean appetizers and snacks incorporate healthy fat sources like olive oil, seeds, and nuts. These fats not only satisfy your hunger and enhance the flavor of the food but also offer significant health benefits, such as improved heart health and reduced inflammation.

1-Hummus Recipe

Time to prepare: 10 minutes

Time to cook: 5 minutes

Serves: 6

Ingredients:

- 1 ½ cups of cooked or canned chickpeas, keep the liquid
- 1 tsp of cumin
- 2 minced garlic cloves
- 1 ½ tbsp of fresh lemon juice
- 2 tbsp of the reserved chickpea liquid
- 4 tbsp of tahini
- 4 tbsp of Greek yogurt
- Pepper and salt to taste

Instructions:

- Combine the chickpeas and all other ingredients in a blender and blend until smooth.
- Transfer the hummus to a serving dish and drizzle with olive oil.
- Serve with fresh vegetables of your choice.

Nutritional Information (Per Serving):

- Calories: 135
- Fat: 6.2 g
- Carbohydrates: 16.3 g

- Sugar: 0.2 g

- Protein: 4.8 g

- Cholesterol: 0 mg

2-Greek Salad Skewers Recipe

Time to prepare: 10 minutes

Time to cook: 10 minutes

Serves: 6

Ingredients:

- 10 pitted olives

- 10 cherry tomatoes

- 1 bell pepper, cored and cut into squares

- ½ a cucumber, cut into half-moon slices

- 6 oz of feta cheese, cubed

For the dressing:

- 1 tsp of dried oregano

- 1 tbsp of olive oil

- 1 tbsp of vinegar

- ½ of fresh lime juice

- 1 tsp of minced garlic

- Pepper and salt to taste

- 12 small 6-inch bamboo skewers

Instructions:

- Thread a cube of cheese, a piece of green pepper, a slice of cucumber, a tomato, and an olive onto each skewer. Repeat with the remaining skewers.

- In a small bowl, mix together the olive oil, garlic, lime juice, vinegar, oregano, pepper, and salt.

- Arrange the skewers on a serving platter and drizzle with the dressing.

- Serve and enjoy.

Nutritional Information (Per Serving):

- Calories: 152

- Fat: 9.7 g

- Carbohydrates: 12.4 g

- Sugar: 8 g

- Protein: 6.3 g

- Cholesterol: 25 mg

3-Grilled Zucchini Roll-Ups Recipe

Time to prepare: 10 minutes

Time to cook: 10 minutes

Serves: 2

Ingredients:

- 3 medium zucchini, sliced lengthwise into ½-inch thick slices

- ½ tsp of fresh lemon juice

- 2 tbsp of chopped fresh basil

- 2 tbsp of chopped fresh parsley

- 4 tbsp of ricotta cheese

- 1 tbsp of olive oil

- Pepper and salt to taste

Instructions:

- Brush the zucchini slices with olive oil on both sides and season with pepper and salt.

- Grill the zucchini slices for about 4 minutes on each side.

- In a small bowl, mix together the cheese, lemon juice, basil, and parsley.

- Spread ½ teaspoon of the cheese mixture onto one end of each zucchini slice, roll up, and place on a serving platter. Repeat with the remaining zucchini slices.

- Serve and enjoy.

Nutritional Information (Per Serving):

- Calories: 152

- Fat: 10 g

- Carbohydrates: 11.8 g

- Sugar: 5.3 g

- Protein: 7.3 g

- Cholesterol: 10 mg

4-Stuffed Grape Leaves Recipe

Time to prepare: 20 minutes

Time to cook: 120 minutes

Serves: 6

Ingredients:

- 1 cup of long-grain white rice, rinsed

- 1 cup of hot water

- ¾ cup of fresh lemon juice

- 4 sprigs of fresh parsley

- 16 oz can of grape leaves

- ½ tsp of ground allspice

- 1 tsp of cinnamon

- ½ cup of pine nuts

- 2 tbsp of chopped mint

- 4 tbsp of chopped parsley

- 2 chopped green onions

- 1 cup of chopped onion

- 1 cup plus 3 tbsp of olive oil

- Pepper and salt to taste

Instructions:

- Heat 3 tablespoons of olive oil in a pan over medium-high heat.

- Add the onion and sauté for 5 minutes.

- Transfer the sautéed onion to a mixing bowl, add the rice, allspice, cinnamon, pine nuts, mint, parsley, green onion, ½ cup of oil, pepper, and salt. Mix well and set aside.

- Rinse the grape leaves and pat dry.

- Place a grape leaf shiny side down on a flat surface.

- Add about 1 tablespoon of the rice mixture to the center of the leaf, fold and roll tightly to form a compact packet. Repeat with the remaining grape leaves and filling.

- Add 2 tablespoons of oil to the bottom of a large pot and cover with a layer of parsley stems.

- Place the stuffed grape leaves on top, drizzle with the remaining olive oil, water, and lemon juice. Top with a plate and a heavy can.

- Cover the pot and bring to a boil, then reduce heat and cook for 1 hour or until the rice is tender.

- Remove from heat and let cool completely.

- Serve and enjoy.

Nutritional Information (Per Serving):

- Calories: 209

- Fat: 8.3 g

- Carbohydrates: 29.7 g

- Sugar: 2.1 g

- Protein: 4.5 g

- Cholesterol: 0 mg

5-Baba Ganoush

Time to Prepare: 10 minutes

Cooking Duration: 40 minutes

Servings: 12

Ingredients:

- 3 medium-sized eggplants, halved lengthwise

- ½ tsp of cumin

- 1 tsp of minced garlic

- 2 tbsp of fresh lemon juice

- 4 tbsp of tahini paste

- 4 tbsp of olive oil

- ¼ tsp of crushed red pepper flakes

- ½ tsp of salt

Instructions:

- Heat the oven to 400 oF.

- Brush the eggplants with 2 tablespoons of olive oil and place them cut side down on a baking sheet lined with parchment paper.

- Bake for 45-50 minutes in the preheated oven until the eggplants are soft.

- After removing from the oven, let them cool completely, then scoop out the flesh of the eggplant and discard the skin.

- Transfer the eggplant flesh and all remaining ingredients, except the red pepper flakes, to a food processor. Blend until the mixture reaches your preferred consistency.

- Drizzle with olive oil and sprinkle with red pepper flakes before serving.

- This dish is best served with vegetables or pita bread.

Nutritional Information (Per Serving):

- Calories: 100

- Fat: 7.6 g

- Carbohydrates: 8 g

- Sugar: 3.5 g

- Protein: 2 g

- Cholesterol: 0 mg

6-Roasted Red Pepper Dip

Time to Prepare: 10 minutes

Cooking Duration: 10 minutes

Servings: 12

Ingredients:

- 16 oz can of drained roasted red peppers

- 1 tbsp of honey

- 1 tbsp of fresh lemon juice

- 1 tbsp of tomato paste

- 1 tsp of smoked paprika

- 1 tsp of ground cumin

- 1 tsp of minced garlic

- ½ cup of diced onion

- 4 tbsp of olive oil

- 1 ½ cups of toasted walnut halves

Instructions:

- Heat 2 tablespoons of olive oil in a pan over medium heat.

- Add the onion to the pan and sauté for 3-5 minutes.

- Add the garlic, tomato paste, paprika, and cumin, and continue cooking for an additional 3-4 minutes.

- Transfer the cooked onion mixture, remaining oil, honey, lemon juice, roasted red peppers, and walnuts to a food processor. Blend until you achieve the desired consistency.

- Serve and enjoy.

Nutritional Information (Per Serving):

- Calories: 80

- Fat: 7.1 g

- Carbohydrates: 5.1 g

- Sugar: 3.2 g

- Protein: 0.9 g

- Cholesterol: 0 mg

7-Caprese Salad

Time to Prepare: 10 minutes

Cooking Duration: 7 minutes

Servings: 4

Ingredients:

- ½ cup of fresh basil

- 1 cup of Bocconcini cheese

- 1 avocado, peeled and chopped into bite-sized pieces

- 5 roasted and quartered Roma tomatoes

- 1 tbsp of olive oil

- 1 tsp of Italian seasoning

- Pepper

- Salt

Instructions:

- Combine the cheese, tomatoes, avocado, basil, oil, Italian seasoning, pepper, and salt in a mixing bowl and toss until well mixed.

- Serve and enjoy.

Nutritional Information (Per Serving):

- Calories: 205

- Fat: 17 g

- Carbohydrates: 10.5 g

- Sugar: 4.4 g

- Protein: 5.4 g

- Cholesterol: 11 mg

8- Tzatziki Sauce

Time to Prepare: 10 minutes

Cooking Duration: 10 minutes

Serves: 8

Ingredients:

- Grated half a large cucumber, ensure to squeeze out the excess liquid

- 1 tablespoon of minced fresh dill

- 1 tablespoon of white vinegar

- 2 tablespoons of olive oil

- 1 teaspoon of minced garlic

- 1 ½ cups of full-fat Greek yogurt

- ½ teaspoon of salt

Steps:

- In a medium-sized bowl, combine the grated cucumber, dill, vinegar, olive oil, garlic, yogurt, and salt and mix well.

- Cover the bowl and refrigerate for 20 minutes.

- Serve chilled and savor the taste.

Nutritional Information (Per Serving):

- Calories: 67

- Fat: 4.1 g

- Carbohydrates: 4.3 g

- Sugar: 3.6 g

- Protein: 2.8 g

- Cholesterol: 3 mg

9- Stuffed Mushrooms with Feta and Spinach

Time to Prepare: 10 minutes

Cooking Duration: 20 minutes

Serves: 4

Ingredients:

- 6 large Portobello mushroom caps, clean out the gills using a spoon

- 1 teaspoon of dried dill

- 1 teaspoon of dried oregano

- 1 teaspoon of grated lemon zest

- 1 cup of crumbled feta cheese

- 6 oz of baby spinach

- 1 teaspoon of minced garlic

- 3 tablespoons of olive oil

- 1 cup of whole wheat bread crumbs

- Pepper

- Salt

Steps:

- Preheat your oven to 475.

- Brush the mushroom caps with olive oil and season with pepper and salt.

- Place the mushroom caps gill side down on a baking sheet and roast in the preheated oven for 10-12 minutes.

- Transfer the mushroom caps to a dish lined with paper to drain.

- In a pan over medium heat, heat 2 tablespoons of olive oil.

- Add garlic, breadcrumbs, pepper, and salt to the pan, stir constantly, and cook for 2-3 minutes.

- Add spinach and cook for 3 minutes or until the spinach wilts. Remove the pan from heat and stir in the dill, oregano, lemon zest, and feta cheese.

- Fill the mushroom caps with the spinach and cheese mixture and place them on a baking sheet lined with parchment paper.

- Return the mushrooms to the oven and roast for 6-8 minutes.

- Serve hot and enjoy.

Nutritional Information (Per Serving):

- Calories: 209

- Fat: 18.8 g

- Carbohydrates: 4.9 g

- Sugar: 2.4 g

- Protein: 7.8 g

- Cholesterol: 33 mg

10- Prosciutto and Melon Skewers

Time to Prepare: 10 minutes

Cooking Duration: 5 minutes

Serves: 6

Ingredients:

- 10 oz of mozzarella pearls, drain excess liquid

- 1 medium-sized cantaloupe

- 10 oz of thin slices of prosciutto crudo

- 12 fresh basil leaves

- 6 10-inch skewers

Steps:

- Cut the cantaloupe in half, remove the seeds, and use a melon baller to scoop out melon balls.

- Assemble one skewer by threading a basil leaf, a melon ball, a slice of prosciutto, and a cheese ball onto it. Repeat the same for the remaining skewers.

- Serve immediately and enjoy.

Nutritional Information (Per Serving):

- Calories: 277

- Fat: 17.1 g

- Carbohydrates: 7.8 g

- Sugar: 7.5 g

- Protein: 21.5 g

- Cholesterol: 42 mg

Salad Recipes

Salads are a fundamental part of the Mediterranean diet, which is renowned for its use of fresh fruits and vegetables. One of the best ways to incorporate a range of nutrient-dense foods into this diet is through salads. These typically include leafy greens such as spinach and lettuce, along with bell peppers, cucumbers, tomatoes, onions, and olives. Mediterranean salads are known for their assortment of colorful vegetables. They are high in fiber, promoting good digestive health and aiding in maintaining a healthy body weight. Consuming these salads can also help lower the risk of chronic illnesses like diabetes, heart disease, and certain cancers.

Olive oil is a key ingredient in Mediterranean salad dressings. It serves as the primary fat source and is rich in healthy monounsaturated fats, offering numerous health advantages. Olive oil is a heart-friendly fat that adds a delicious flavor and richness to your salad. It is also a concentrated source of essential vitamins, minerals, and antioxidants. Salads are versatile and can be easily tailored to individual tastes and preferences. They can be made with various combinations of fruits, vegetables, nuts, seeds, whole grains, and lean proteins like grilled fish or chicken, allowing for a wide range of flavors and textures in the Mediterranean diet.

Salads are low in calories and can help manage body weight. They provide satisfying and filling meal options without excessive calorie intake, making them an excellent choice for those aiming to maintain a healthy weight. Mediterranean salads, with their mix of herbs, colorful vegetables, and spices, are rich in antioxidants. These antioxidants help protect against inflammation, reduce oxidative stress, and lower the risk of chronic diseases.

1- Greek Salad Recipe

Ready in: 15 minutes

Serves: 6

Ingredients:

For the salad:

- ½ cup of pitted kalamata olives

- 1 small onion, sliced

- 5 tomatoes, cut into 1-inch pieces

- 1 cucumber, peeled and cut into 1-inch pieces

- 1 green bell pepper, cut into 1-inch pieces

- 8 oz of feta cheese, cut into ½-inch pieces

For the dressing:

- 1/3 cup of olive oil

- 1 tsp of dried dill

- 1 ½ tsp of dried oregano

- 1 tsp of minced garlic

- 4 tbsp of red wine vinegar

- Pepper and salt to taste

Instructions:

- Combine all the dressing ingredients in a small bowl and set it aside.

- In a large bowl, mix the olives, onion, tomatoes, cucumber, bell pepper, and feta cheese.

- Pour the dressing over the salad and mix well.

- Serve immediately and enjoy.

Nutritional Information (Per Serving):

- Calories: 250

- Fat: 20.8g

- Carbohydrates: 11.2g

- Sugar: 6.6g

- Protein: 7.1g

- Cholesterol: 34mg

2- Caprese Salad Recipe

Ready in: 15 minutes

Serves: 6

Ingredients:

- 1 cup of mozzarella balls

- ¼ cup of chopped fresh basil

- ¼ tsp of dried thyme

- 2 tbsp of balsamic vinegar

- 2 tbsp of olive oil

- 2 cups of cherry tomatoes, halved

- Pepper and salt to taste

Instructions:

- In a large bowl, combine the tomatoes, basil, and mozzarella balls.

- In a small bowl, whisk together the olive oil, thyme, vinegar, pepper, and salt.

- Pour the dressing over the tomato mixture and mix well.

- Cover and refrigerate until ready to serve.

Nutritional Information (Per Serving):

- Calories: 66

- Fat: 5.6g

- Carbohydrates: 2.6g

- Sugar: 1.6g

- Protein: 1.9g

- Cholesterol: 3mg

3- Tuna and Bean Salad Recipe

Ready in: 15 minutes

Serves: 8

Ingredients:

- 10 oz of albacore tuna in olive oil

- Juice of ½ a lemon

- ¼ cup of chopped fresh parsley

- ¾ cup of crumbled feta cheese

- ½ cup of julienned sun-dried tomatoes

- ½ cup of chopped kalamata olives

- 1 medium onion, chopped

- 15.5 oz can of great northern beans, drained and rinsed

- Pepper and salt to taste

Instructions:

- Combine the tuna and all the other ingredients in a large bowl and mix well.

- Serve immediately or refrigerate for 1 hour before serving.

Nutritional Information (Per Serving):

- Calories: 200

- Fat: 9.2g

- Carbohydrates: 14.5g

- Sugar: 1.5g

- Protein: 14.7g

- Cholesterol: 25mg

4-Chickpea Salad

This recipe takes 10 minutes to prepare and 5 minutes to cook. It serves 4 people.

Ingredients:

- One 30 oz can of chickpeas, drained and rinsed

- ¼ cup of crumbled feta cheese

- ½ cup of pitted kalamata olives

- 4 tablespoons of fresh chopped basil

- 4 tablespoons of fresh chopped parsley

- 1 cup of halved cherry tomatoes

- 1 cup of diced cucumber

- 1 medium chopped onion

- 1 chopped bell pepper

For the dressing:

- 3 tablespoons of olive oil
- ½ teaspoon of red pepper flakes
- 1 teaspoon of minced garlic
- 2 tablespoons of fresh lemon juice
- 2 tablespoons of red wine vinegar
- Pepper and salt to taste

Directions:

- Combine chickpeas, feta cheese, olives, basil, parsley, tomatoes, cucumber, onion, and bell pepper in a large bowl.
- In a small bowl, whisk together all the dressing ingredients and pour over the salad.
- Mix well and serve.

Nutritional Value (Per Serving):

- Calories: 427
- Fat: 17.1g
- Carbohydrates: 57.9g
- Sugar: 4.9g
- Protein: 13.5g
- Cholesterol: 8mg

5-Quinoa Salad

This recipe takes 10 minutes to prepare and 10 minutes to cook. It serves 4 people.

Ingredients:

For the salad:

- 2 cups of cooked quinoa

- 4 tablespoons of crumbled feta cheese

- ½ cup of chopped fresh basil

- 4 tablespoons of chopped sun-dried tomatoes

- ½ cup of halved kalamata olives

- ½ a small chopped onion

- 1 cup of cooked chickpeas

- ½ a chopped cucumber

- 1 chopped bell pepper

For the dressing:

- 1/3 cup of olive oil

- ¼ teaspoon of ground cumin

- ½ teaspoon of garlic powder

- ½ teaspoon of dried oregano

- 1 teaspoon of honey

- 1 tablespoon of Dijon mustard

- 1 tablespoon of red wine vinegar

- 2 tablespoons of fresh lemon juice

- Pepper and salt to taste

Directions:

- Mix all salad ingredients in a large bowl.

- In a small bowl, whisk together all the dressing ingredients and pour over the salad.

- Toss well and serve.

Nutritional Value (Per Serving):

- Calories: 717

- Fat: 29.2g

- Carbohydrates: 93.6g

- Sugar: 10.3g

- Protein: 24.3g

- Cholesterol: 8mg

6-Tabouli Salad

This recipe takes 10 minutes to prepare and 10 minutes to cook. It serves 6 people.

Ingredients:

- ½ cup of bulgur wheat

- ¼ cup of olive oil

- Juice of ½ a lemon

- 4 chopped green onions

- ¼ cup of chopped fresh mint

- 2 bunches of chopped parsley

- 1 chopped cucumber

- 4 chopped tomatoes

- Pepper and salt to taste

Directions:

- Rinse the bulgur wheat and soak it in water for 5 minutes. Drain well and set aside.

- In a bowl, combine the bulgur, green onions, mint, parsley, cucumber, and tomatoes.

- In a separate bowl, mix the olive oil, lemon juice, pepper, and salt. Pour this mixture over the bulgur mixture and mix well. Cover and refrigerate for 30 minutes.

- Serve and enjoy.

Nutritional Value (Per Serving):

- Calories: 139

- Fat: 8.8g

- Carbohydrates: 14.9g

- Sugar: 3.3g

- Protein: 2.8g

- Cholesterol: 0mg

7- Caesar Salad Recipe

Time to Prepare: 10 minutes

Cooking Duration: 10 minutes

Serves: 4 people

Ingredients Required:

- 2 chicken breasts, cooked and sliced into strips

- ¼ cup of croutons

- 1/3 cup of grated parmesan cheese

- 1 large chopped romaine lettuce

- For the dressing:

- 1 cup of homemade olive oil mayonnaise

- ½ cup of grated parmesan cheese

- 1 tsp of Worcestershire sauce

- 1 tsp of Dijon mustard

- 2 tbsp of fresh lemon juice

- 1 tsp of anchovy paste

- 1 tsp of minced garlic

- Pepper and Salt to taste

Instructions:

- Combine all the dressing ingredients in a small bowl and keep it aside.

- Place the lettuce in a serving bowl, sprinkle parmesan cheese, add croutons and chicken.

- Pour the dressing over the salad and toss gently until it's well mixed.

- Serve immediately and enjoy.

Nutritional Value (Per Serving):

- Calories: 455

- Fat: 31 g

- Carbohydrates: 16 g

- Sugar: 4 g

- Protein: 30 g

- Cholesterol: 101 mg

8- Waldorf Salad Recipe

Time to Prepare: 10 minutes

Cooking Duration: 10 minutes

Serves: 4 people

Ingredients Required:

- 2 apples, cored and cubed

- 2 tbsp of fresh lemon juice

- ½ cup of Greek yogurt

- 2 tbsp of chopped walnuts

- ½ cup of diced celery

- 2/3 cup of seedless grapes

- 1 pear, cored and cubed

Instructions:

- In a mixing bowl, combine yogurt and lemon juice.

- Add apples, walnuts, celery, grapes, and pear, and mix everything well until well coated.

- Cover the salad and refrigerate for 30 minutes before serving.

- Serve chilled and enjoy.

Nutritional Value (Per Serving):

- Calories: 138

- Fat: 3.1 g

- Carbohydrates: 26.4 g

- Sugar: 20 g

- Protein: 3.4 g

- Cholesterol: 2 mg

9- Beet and Goat Cheese Salad Recipe

Time to Prepare: 10 minutes

Cooking Duration: 5 minutes

Serves: 4 people

Ingredients Required:

- For the salad:

- 2 cups of arugula

- 2 cups of chopped spinach

- ¼ cup of crumbled feta cheese

- 1/3 cup of chopped pecans

- 1 small sliced onion

- 1 cup of chopped roasted beets

- For the dressing:

- ¼ cup of olive oil

- ¼ cup of apple cider vinegar

- 4 tbsp of brown sugar

Instructions:

- Combine olive oil, vinegar, and brown sugar in a small bowl and keep it aside.
- In a serving bowl, layer arugula and spinach, followed by beets, onion, pecans, and cheese.
- Drizzle the dressing over the salad and serve.

Nutritional Value (Per Serving):

- Calories: 198
- Fat: 15 g
- Carbohydrates: 14 g
- Sugar: 10 g
- Protein: 2 g
- Cholesterol: 9 mg

10- Shrimp and Avocado Salad Recipe

Time to Prepare: 10 minutes

Cooking Duration: 10 minutes

Serves: 4 people

Ingredients Required:

- 1 lb of cooked shrimp
- 4 oz of toasted sliced almonds
- 1 minced shallot
- 1 diced avocado
- ½ lemon juice
- 2 tbsp of olive oil
- 4 cups of arugula
- 4 cups of spinach

- Pepper and Salt to taste

Instructions:

- In a mixing bowl, combine shrimp, almonds, shallot, avocado, arugula, and spinach.

- Mix olive oil, lemon juice, pepper, and salt and pour over the salad.

- Toss the salad well and serve.

Nutritional Value (Per Serving):

- Calories: 473

- Fat: 33 g

- Carbohydrates: 14 g

- Sugar: 2 g

- Protein: 34 g

- Cholesterol: 239 mg

Main Dish Recipes

The centerpiece of the Mediterranean diet is the main course, which is a combination of various nutrient-dense foods. This diet is well-known for its focus on the main course, which is a balanced and nutritious mix of different food groups. The main course in the Mediterranean diet is carefully crafted to offer a balanced mix of macronutrients such as proteins, fats, carbohydrates, and various essential micronutrients. It typically includes a generous portion of vegetables, lean protein from sources like fish, poultry, legumes, or eggs, whole grains, and healthy fats from seeds, nuts, and olive oil. This blend of all the necessary and healthy nutrients makes it a quintessential Mediterranean dish.

The Mediterranean diet emphasizes the consumption of plant-based foods, and the main course is no exception. It usually includes a variety of vegetables, whole grains, legumes, herbs, and spices. These plant-based foods and ingredients are loaded with essential vitamins, minerals, antioxidants, and fiber. Olive oil, a primary source of monounsaturated fats, is frequently used in the Mediterranean diet. It enhances the flavor and richness of the main course while also promoting heart health and reducing the risk of cardiovascular disease.

Mediterranean cuisine is renowned for its use of herbs and spices that add flavor to dishes. The main course in the Mediterranean diet often includes a variety of herbs and spices such as oregano, basil, rosemary, thyme, cumin, and garlic. These herbs and spices not only enhance the flavor of the main course but also offer potential health benefits. In Mediterranean culture, meals are often considered social and cultural events where friends and family gather to enjoy a shared meal.

1- Lemon Garlic Shrimp Recipe

Preparation Time: 10 minutes

Cooking Time: 5 minutes

Serves: 4

Ingredients:

- 1 lb of peeled and deveined shrimp
- 3 tbsp of chopped fresh parsley
- 2 tbsp of fresh lemon juice
- 4 minced garlic cloves
- 1 tbsp of olive oil
- Pepper
- Salt

Instructions:

- Mix shrimp with pepper and salt in a bowl.
- Heat oil in a pan over medium heat.
- Sauté garlic for 30 seconds.
- Add shrimp to the pan and cook for 2 minutes.
- Flip the shrimp, add lemon juice, and cook for another 2 minutes or until fully cooked.
- Mix in parsley.
- Serve immediately and enjoy.

Nutritional Value (Per Serving):

- Calories: 172
- Fat: 5 g
- Carbohydrates: 3 g
- Sugar: 0.2 g
- Protein: 26.2 g
- Cholesterol: 239 mg

2- Chicken and Vegetable Skewers Recipe

Preparation Time: 10 minutes

Cooking Time: 10 minutes

Serves: 6

Ingredients:

- 1 large onion, cut into 1 ½-inch pieces
- 2 medium zucchini, sliced
- 2 bell peppers, cut into 1 ½-inch pieces
- 1 lb boneless chicken breast, cut into 1 ½-inch pieces
- 2 tbsp of chopped fresh parsley
- 2 tbsp of chopped fresh dill
- 1 tsp of minced garlic
- ½ cup of fresh lemon juice
- ½ cup of olive oil
- Pepper
- Salt

Instructions:

- Whisk together oil, garlic, lemon juice, parsley, dill, pepper, and salt in a small bowl. Set aside.

- Thread chicken and vegetables onto pre-soaked wooden skewers.

- Place skewers in a casserole dish, then pour marinade over them. Cover and refrigerate for 40 minutes.

- Preheat the grill to medium heat.

- Grill marinated chicken and vegetable skewers for 5-8 minutes on each side or until the chicken is fully cooked.

- Serve and enjoy.

Nutritional Value (Per Serving):

- Calories: 272

- Fat: 19 g

- Carbohydrates: 8 g

- Sugar: 4 g

- Protein: 17 g

- Cholesterol: 48 mg

3- Greek Salad with Grilled Chicken Recipe

Preparation Time: 10 minutes

Cooking Time: 15 minutes

Serves: 4

Ingredients:

For the chicken:

- 1 lb chicken tenders

- 1 tbsp minced garlic

- 1 tbsp Montreal grill seasoning

- 1 tbsp ground coriander

- 1 tbsp smoked paprika

- 1 tbsp cumin

- 1 tbsp chili powder

- 1 tbsp olive oil

- Juice of 1 lemon

- 1 tsp salt

For the salad:

- ½ cup crumbled feta cheese

- ½ cup chopped cucumber

- ¼ cup chopped pepperoncini peppers

- ¼ cup pitted kalamata olives

- ½ cup sliced cherry tomatoes

- 1 head of romaine lettuce

For the dressing:

- 4 tbsp olive oil

- 1 tbsp Greek seasoning

- ¼ cup red wine vinegar

Instructions:

- In a large bowl, combine chicken, oil, and spices. Rub mixture all over the chicken. Cover and refrigerate for 4 hours.

- Preheat the grill to medium heat.

- Grill marinated chicken for 4-5 minutes. Flip and cook for an additional 3 minutes or until fully cooked.

- In a separate bowl, combine all salad ingredients. Top with grilled chicken.

- In a small bowl, whisk together all dressing ingredients and drizzle over chicken and salad.

- Serve and enjoy.

Nutritional Value (Per Serving):

- Calories: 470

- Fat: 32 g

- Carbohydrates: 9 g

- Sugar: 2.9 g

- Protein: 37 g

- Cholesterol: 118 mg

4. Pasta with Roasted Eggplant and Tomato

Preparation: 10 minutes

Cooking: 25 minutes

Servings: 6

Ingredients:

- 10 oz of long pasta

For the vegetables:

- 1 medium-sized eggplant, cut into cubes

- 2 cups of cherry tomatoes

- 2 cloves of garlic

- Pepper and salt to taste

For the sauce:

- 3 tablespoons of olive oil

- 1/2 cup of fresh basil

- 1/2 cup of marinated artichoke hearts, chopped

- 1/4 cup of halved kalamata olives

- 2 cloves of garlic, sliced

- 1/3 cup of diced onion

Instructions:

1. Cook the pasta as per the instructions on the package, then drain and set aside.

2. Preheat your oven to 450°F.

3. On a baking sheet lined with parchment paper, spread out the tomatoes, eggplant, and garlic. Season with pepper and salt.

4. Roast the vegetables in the preheated oven for 20 minutes, stirring halfway through.

5. For the sauce: In a pan, heat the oil over medium heat.

6. Add the garlic and onion to the pan and sauté until the onions are soft. Add the tomatoes, eggplant, olives, garlic, and artichoke, then stir well.

7. Add the cooked pasta and basil to the pan and toss everything together until well coated.

8. Serve and enjoy.

Nutritional Information (Per Serving):

- Calories: 299

- Fat: 10.2g

- Carbohydrates: 44.9g

- Sugar: 6g

- Protein: 7.9g

- Cholesterol: 0mg

5. Salmon Baked with Herbed Yogurt Sauce

Preparation: 10 minutes

Cooking: 20 minutes

Servings: 4

Ingredients:

- 1 lb boneless salmon fillet

- 1 tablespoon of honey

- 1 tablespoon of drained and chopped capers

- 2 tablespoons of chopped dill

- 2 tablespoons of chopped mint

- 1/4 cup of chopped parsley

- 1 tablespoon of Dijon mustard

- 1/2 cup of Greek yogurt

- Pepper and salt to taste

Instructions:

1. Preheat your oven to 350°F.

2. Place the salmon on a baking sheet lined with parchment paper. Season the salmon with pepper and salt.

3. In a bowl, combine the yogurt, honey, capers, herbs, mustard, pepper, and salt until well mixed.

4. Spread the yogurt mixture evenly over the salmon.

5. Bake the salmon in the preheated oven for 15-20 minutes.

6. Serve and enjoy.

Nutritional Information (Per Serving):

- Calories: 176

- Fat: 7.3g

- Carbohydrates: 6g

- Sugar: 4g

- Protein: 22g

- Cholesterol: 50mg

Dessert Recipes

Mediterranean diet desserts are typically savored sparingly and are often associated with special occasions or celebrations rather than being a daily indulgence. The diet encourages moderate consumption by advocating for smaller dessert portions. Instead of large servings of rich, sugary treats, the focus is on savoring smaller portions made from nutritious ingredients. This approach allows one to satisfy a sweet tooth without overloading on calories. Fresh fruit, a staple of the Mediterranean diet, is often used as a healthier alternative to traditional high-sugar desserts. These fruits provide natural sweetness and are packed with vitamins, minerals, and fiber. They can be enjoyed on their own or incorporated into simple fruit-based desserts.

Mediterranean diet desserts often feature a blend of nutrient-dense ingredients like fresh fruits, seeds, nuts, whole grains, and yogurt. These ingredients not only add to the flavor but also increase the nutritional value of the dessert by providing additional vitamins, minerals, fiber, and antioxidants. The Mediterranean diet encourages homemade desserts over processed or packaged ones. Making desserts at home allows for better control over the ingredients used, their quality, and the amount of sugar added. It also provides an opportunity to experiment with healthier ingredients and make adjustments based on individual needs.

The Mediterranean diet emphasizes overall nutritional balance and diversity. Desserts are not the main focus of the diet, but enjoying a sweet treat occasionally adds to the enjoyment and satisfaction derived from this eating pattern. It's still crucial to monitor overall calorie intake and balance it with a variety of nutrient-rich whole foods in your meals. By choosing healthier dessert options, one can indulge a sweet craving while still adhering to the principles of the Mediterranean diet.

1- Honey and Walnut Greek Yogurt

Preparation Time: 5 minutes

Cooking Time: 5 minutes

Serves: 2

Ingredients:

- 2 tbsp of toasted and chopped walnuts

- 1/4 cup of honey

- 2 cups of Greek yogurt

Instructions:

- In a small bowl, blend the honey and walnuts.

- Split the yogurt into two serving glasses and garnish with the honey walnut mixture.

- Ready to serve and enjoy.

Nutritional Value (Per Serving):

- Calories: 351

- Fat: 7 g

- Carbohydrates: 52 g

- Sugar: 52 g

- Protein: 16 g

- Cholesterol: 15 mg

2- Refreshing Fruit Salad

Preparation Time: 10 minutes

Cooking Time: 5 minutes

Serves: 8

Ingredients:

For the salad:

- 2 peeled and sliced bananas

- 1 cup of fresh raspberries

- 1 cup of blueberries

- 1 peeled, cored, and diced apple

- 2 segmented and diced oranges

- 4 cups of sliced fresh strawberries

For the dressing:

- 1 ½ cups of Greek yogurt

- 3 tbsp of honey

- 1 /2 of orange juice

Instructions:

- In a mixing bowl, combine strawberries, oranges, apples, blueberries, raspberries, and bananas.

- In another small bowl, whisk together the yogurt, orange juice, and honey. Drizzle this dressing over the salad and mix well.

- Ready to serve and enjoy.

Nutritional Value (Per Serving):

- Calories: 163

- Fat: 1.2 g

- Carbohydrates: 36 g

- Sugar: 27 g

- Protein: 4 g

- Cholesterol: 3 mg

3- Almond Flour Cookies

Preparation Time: 10 minutes

Cooking Time: 10 minutes

Serves: 6

Ingredients:

- 1 cup of almond flour

- ½ tsp of almond extract

- ¼ tsp of vanilla

- 2 tbsp of chopped almonds

- 5 tbsp of maple syrup

Instructions:

- Preheat the oven to 350 oF.

- In a mixing bowl, combine almond flour, almond extract, vanilla, almonds, and maple syrup until a dough forms.

- Form equal-sized balls from the almond flour mixture.

- Flatten each dough ball and place it on a baking sheet lined with parchment paper.

- Bake in the preheated oven for 10-12 minutes or until the cookies turn a light golden brown.

- Remove the cookies from the oven and let them cool completely.

- Ready to serve and enjoy.

Nutritional Value (Per Serving):

- Calories: 163

- Fat: 10.4 g

- Carbohydrates: 15 g

- Sugar: 10 g

- Protein: 4 g

- Cholesterol: 0 mg

Recipe 4: Honey and Cinnamon Baked Pears

Preparation Time: 10 minutes

Cooking Time: 30 minutes

Serves: 4

Ingredients:

- 4 medium-sized pears, peeled, cored, and halved

- ½ teaspoon of vanilla

- ½ teaspoon of cinnamon

- 2 tablespoons of coconut oil

- 3 tablespoons of honey

Instructions:

- Preheat your oven to 400 degrees Fahrenheit.

- Place the pears in a baking dish.

- Combine honey, vanilla, coconut oil, and cinnamon in a microwave-safe bowl and heat for 30 seconds. Stir until well mixed.

- Drizzle the honey mixture over the pears and bake in the preheated oven for 30 minutes.

- Remove from the oven and let it cool completely.

- Serve and enjoy.

Nutritional Value (Per Serving):

- Calories: 205

- Fat: 7g

- Carbohydrates: 38g

- Sugar: 29g

- Protein: 0.7g

- Cholesterol: 0mg

Recipe 5: Strawberries Dipped in Dark Chocolate

Preparation Time: 10 minutes

Cooking Time: 10 minutes

Serves: 4

Ingredients:

- 12 medium-sized fresh strawberries, washed and dried

* 1 teaspoon of avocado oil

* 3 ounces of chopped dark chocolate

Instructions:

* Prepare a plate lined with parchment paper.

* Put the chopped chocolate in a microwave-safe bowl and heat for 1 minute, stirring every 30 seconds.

* Remove the melted chocolate from the microwave.

* Add avocado oil to the melted chocolate and stir until well mixed.

* Dip each strawberry into the melted chocolate, allowing any excess to drip off.

* Place the chocolate-covered strawberries on the prepared plate and refrigerate for 30 minutes.

* Serve and enjoy.

Nutritional Value (Per Serving):

* Calories: 127

* Fat: 6g

* Carbohydrates: 15g

* Sugar: 12g

* Protein: 1.9g

* Cholesterol: 5mg

Conclusion

Thank you for taking the time to read this book to the end. I hope you found it enlightening and full of useful tools to help you achieve your health goals.

By engaging with this book, you've taken a crucial initial step on an exciting journey towards improved health and a fresh, new perspective on food. You now possess the secret to the long, healthy and joyful lives led by many people in the Mediterranean region, surrounded by their loved ones. So, what's your next move now that you're privy to this secret?

Your next step is to put on your chef's hat and start cooking! Begin your grocery shopping and cooking as soon as you can. You're probably eager to try out some of the mouth-watering recipes you came across in this guide. If you need further assistance, there's a vast community of people online and around your local area who have also adopted the Mediterranean lifestyle. They are ready and willing to support you as you delve into this new dietary and lifestyle approach. Don't forget to put on your walking shoes and start being physically active from today. The sooner you begin, the quicker you'll reach your goals of creating and maintaining a healthier lifestyle. You're at an exciting new stage in your life, so savor every moment!

Lastly, if you found this book beneficial in any way, I would greatly appreciate a review on Amazon.